AIDS and American Apocalypticism

SUNY series in the Sociology of Culture

Charles R. Simpson, editor

AIDS and American Apocalypticism

The Cultural Semiotics of an Epidemic

DISCARD

Thomas L. Long

STATE UNIVERSITY OF NEW YORK PRESS

Published by
State University of New York Press, Albany

For information, address State University of New York Press,
194 Washington Avenue, Suite 305, Albany, NY 12210-2365

Production by Michael Haggett
Marketing by Susan M. Petrie

Library of Congress Cataloging-in-Publication Data

Long, Thomas L.
    AIDS and American apocalypticism : the cultural semiotics of an epidemic /
Thomas L. Long.
        p. cm. — (SUNY series in the sociology of culture)
    Includes bibliographical references and index.
    ISBN 0-7914-6167-X (alk. paper) — ISBN 0-7914-6168-8 (pbk. : alk. paper)
    1. AIDS (Disease)—United States—Religious aspects. 2. Apocalyptic literature.
I. Title. II. Series.
    [DNLM: 1. Acquired Immunodeficiency Syndrome—psychology. 2. Religion
and Medicine. 3. Medicine in Literature. 4. Morals. 5. Public Opinion.
WC 503.7 L849a 2004]
RA643.83.L66 2004
362.196'9792'00973—dc22   2004022402

10 9 8 7 6 5 4 3 2 1

To my parents

In memory of

Jack	Kerry	Tim	Charley	Andy	Brett
Ray	Jerry	Jack	Sonny	Doug	Mike
Andy	Jack	Glynn	Roger	Tim	Jack
Bill	Mike	Rusty	Reilly	Jim	Patrick
	Harvey	Bill	Virgil	Michael	

and the others whose names I have forgotten.

Si lunga tratta
di gente, ch'io non avrei mai creduto
che morte tanta n'avesse disfatta. Inferno III, 55–57
("I had not thought death had undone so many")

Contents

Preface

This book grew out of rage and grief, my own, of course, but also that of others. During the 1980s as a Roman Catholic priest, I struggled with the awful and initially limited knowledge of an epidemic, first called "Gay Related Immune Dysfunction" (GRID), later Acquired Immunodeficiency Syndrome (AIDS). At the hospital bedside of sick and dying people, beside their families, friends, lovers at funerals, and in the horrible solitude of my own room where I read my body daily for any signifier of disease, I was confronted by the human need to make sense of this epidemic. During the 1990s and now, as an academic, activist, and public intellectual, I have wrestled with the purposes of social and cultural analysis in the midst of a public health crisis. One result is this book.

A book is not written so much as it is built, and this book, as much as most, relied on a large construction crew. Michael Vella, professor of American Studies at Indiana University of Pennsylvania, who served as my mentor in this book's early life, provided caring and careful critiques of it at every stage. Patrick Murphy, in the English Department of Central Florida University, and Cecilia Rodríguez-Milanés, director of Women's Studies at Central Florida University, provided searching questions that led to its further improvement. Anonymous reviewers and series editor, Charles Simpson, for the State University of New York Press afforded me what every writer desires: a sympathetic, careful, and critically fair reading, with recommendations for revisions.

John T. Dever, my former Communications and Humanities Division dean at Thomas Nelson Community College and now executive vice president of Northern Virginia Community College, has been both an inspiration and a mentor. Educational leave provided by Thomas Nelson Community College permitted me seven uninterrupted months to research and write.

The members of the monthly Gay Men's Book Group of Hampton Roads (Virginia) have been encouraging friends and alert readers, and I am particularly grateful to Lee Hanson, Kirk Read, Charles Rhodes, and Charles Ford for their comments on drafts.

My hosts in New York City, the Franciscan Friars of the Atonement, made it possible for me to spend weeks and months for several years doing research in the city. My longtime friends, Rev. James Gardiner, SA and Rev. Joe Cavoto, SA, have provided me with ideas and contacts. Laurence Pagnoni has also been a guide and patron in the city. Those with whom I conducted interviews generously shared their time and lives, among them Douglas Petitjean, the late Keith Christopher, Ishmael Houston-Jones, Steed Taylor, Tim Miller, and Samuel R. Delany. Many Internet correspondents replied to my e-mail queries to Listserv groups.

My best "bud" John Elliott has always encouraged me to run the race to the end. My psychiatrist, Howard Weiss, M.D., provided good counsel and good meds. Dr. Michael Schiefelbein, professor of English at Christian Brothers University in Memphis, Tennessee, provided guidance and encouragement at a critical juncture that helped me bring this book to publication. Dr. George Greenia of the College of William and Mary injected me with his enthusiasm as needed.

Several research institutions have been invaluable in this study. The library of Regent University, the institution founded in Virginia Beach by televangelist Pat Robertson, was, not surprisingly, a trove of fundamentalist discourse on homosexuality and AIDS; and, like most libraries, it was also admirably stocked with work by gay writers and postmodern critical theorists. "Know your enemy" cuts both ways. Local research libraries at Old Dominion University and the College of William and Mary provided both reference and source materials. The New York Public Library has been invaluable in research for this study, in particular the Main Reading Room staff and the librarians of the Miriam and Ira D. Wallach Division of Art, Prints and Photographs room at the Central Research Library, and the staff of the New York Public Library for the Performing Arts at Lincoln Center, particularly those in the Theatre on Film and Tape Archive. I am especially indebted to the National Archive of Lesbian and Gay History, whose staff (Richard C. Wandel, archivist and Nancy D. Seaton, project archivist) and volunteers made me feel at home and supported my work in more ways than I can count.

My greatest debt, however, is to my parents, Thomas Lawrence Long, Sr. and Lucy McVey Long, who believed in this work, and without whom it would not have been completed.

Chapter One

Apocalyptus Interruptus
Christianity, Sodomy, and the End

Walking out of the library of Regent University in Virginia Beach, Virginia, the private Christian fundamentalist school founded in 1977 by televangelist and onetime Republican presidential hopeful Pat Robertson, students and visitors are confronted by a monumental stone and welded-steel sculpture of the Four Horsemen of the Apocalypse by Cyd Chambers Players. The sculpture's terrifying subject strikes a contrast to the meticulously landscaped campus with its elegant neo-Georgian brick architecture: Ivy League Doomsday. The apparent contradiction of two styles—nostalgic idealization of the Early Republic and urgent expectation of the end-time—aptly represents the paradox and the persuasiveness of American apocalypticism. The son of a United States senator and an alumnus of Yale, Robertson has built a communications empire, beginning with his flagship daily television program, *The 700 Club*, by providing his electronic flock with prophetic interpretations of current events and with oracular utterances warning of God's imminent wrath. His personal wealth and the sophistication of his business, educational, and philanthropic operations should put to rest the notion that apocalyptic or millennialist beliefs are the sign of the clinically delusional or of rural snake-handlers. Indeed, many Americans believe that the nation is poised on the brink—of the abyss or of the new age or of both. In the last two decades of the twentieth century, AIDS and American homosexuals would preoccupy their apocalyptic fantasies.

In 1981 the headlines "Disease Rumors Largely Unfounded" and "Rare Cancer Seen in 41 Homosexuals" (the first reports of what would eventually be called "AIDS"), entered a cluttered discursive landscape. The rhetoric of American religious conservatives in the late 1970s—most visibly the political action group "Moral Majority" and television evangelists like Pat Robertson and Jerry Falwell—had already constructed homosexuality itself as a contagious disease and as an apocalyptic signifier, a sign of the "end times."[1] During the first AIDS decade, the coincidence of male homosexuality with a hideously fatal infectious agent intensified this apocalyptic rhetoric, not only among Christian fundamentalists but also within those groups most affected by AIDS. Throughout the 1980s and into the second decade of the epidemic, HIV/AIDS affected/infected culture workers attempted to wrest control of hostile apocalyptic images by appropriating them for their own purposes. That two opposed groups in American cultural politics could each employ the same tropes for competing ideological purposes attests both to the pervasiveness of apocalypticism in American culture and to the resilience of its signs. This book will draft a map of that discursive landscape on which AIDS partisans conducted their forays equally against the social effects of the medical syndrome and against the religious rhetoric employed to stigmatize the syndrome and those affected by it. The purpose of this study is to provide both an account and a critique of apocalyptic discourse on behalf of the HIV/AIDS affected/infected through a historicist social semiotic analysis of various discursive forms: fiction, drama, performance art, mixed media art, video, film, graphics, journalism, and biomedical discourse and will examine four salient apocalyptic tropes: exile, the prophetic utterance known as the jeremiad, sacred warfare or Armageddon, and paradisal bliss.

FUNDAMENTALISM, SODOMY, AND APOCALYPTICISM

In the second half of the 1970s religious conservatives in the United States began to consolidate their cultural and political power around the diffuse social anxieties of "middle Americans" who had been characterized earlier in the decade as a "silent majority." Among the "hot button" issues were gender and sexuality, particularly in the forms of North American feminism and gay rights activism. White males increasingly perceived themselves as competing for dwindling economic power with women as well as with people of other races and ethnicities. A more visible and vocal gay and lesbian activism, then increasingly supported by some progressive politicians and religious leaders, began to make inroads into local and national politics. Christian fundamentalists, already politically conservative and increasingly allied with monied interests, began to oppose one particular strain of progressivism—activism for gay and lesbian equal rights.

Nowhere was this reaction more evident than in Anita Bryant's nationally publicized 1977 campaign to repeal the Dade County, Florida, gay equal rights ordinance. In her own account of the "Save Our Children" campaign—initially unsuccessful, but eventually effective in repealing the ordinance through a public referendum—Bryant recalled a conversation with her pastor, William Chapman, after the ordinance was first passed by the Metro Dade Commission:

> Brother Bill stopped whistling and looked at us and said, "You know what it is?" He paused, noticing that we were finally relaxing. "God has given us *a space to repent.*" "How do you know that?" I asked him. "Revelation, chapter 2, verse 21. The writer had been describing the wicked prophetess Jezebel, and then he says: 'And I gave her space to repent of her fornication; and she repented not.' Remember, the Book of Revelation is a book of prophecy. America is being given time—a space to repent. . . . One of two things will come to pass, Anita. . . . There will be revival or ruin."[2]

"Brother Bill"'s reading of the "signs of the times," events leading for some to a crisis of identity and meaning, is characteristic in two respects: homosexuality is read as a harbinger of catastrophe, even the ultimate catastrophe, and the present moment is figured as a binary opposition or crisis—revival or ruin. Bryant had apparently perceived the latter (the campaign after all was to "Save Our Children") and had begun to elaborate on the former. In her remarks on *The PTL Club*, televangelist Jim Bakker's daily program, Bryant offered this historical exegesis:

> We know that the once-powerful Roman Empire gradually rotted from within and fell to barbarian invaders; just so, our civilization is headed for destruction unless we change our present course. We felt that we had to take a stand along with other concerned Miamians. We are faced with an aggressive social *epidemic* [emphasis mine] in this country, but, praise God, I do believe in the decency of the American people, and I believe this downward trend can be reversed . . .

Later that month she would appear with a similar message on Pat Robertson's daily television program, *The 700 Club*.[3] Homosexuality was thus imagined as a plague-like epidemic threatening the entire American body.

While Bryant may have been one of the most visible proponents of the view that homosexuality is a precursor of a society's collapse or apocalypse, she was by no means its sole advocate. In the previous decade, Israel's successful capture of the city of Jerusalem in the 1967 Six-Days War prompted renewed Christian fundamentalist apocalyptic speculations. Well over a thousand international delegates, among them Anita Bryant and C. Everett Koop, the future Reagan-appointed Surgeon General when AIDS was first identified, met in the Holy City for a 1971 prophecy conference. One of the speakers at the conference, Harold John Ockenga, compared his time in history with that of the biblical Noah, but contended that the modern world was even more ripe for apocalyptic destruction:

> Here, in addition to the conditions of the days of Noah, we have perversions of sex, including sodomy, homosexuality and Lesbianism. Strange as it may seem, these movements have now come out in the open, are demanding recognition in society as legitimate, and are being portrayed for us on the screen and in the theater. Many people are turning to sexual perversion.

Ockenga cited the years 1965 to 1970 as having been a particular turning point in the West's decline. Another conference speaker, Wilbur Smith, related changing sexual attitudes to Jesus' prophecy about the end times:

> There is one aspect of this present lawlessness which I believe for the first time in modern history relates world conditions to a certain prophecy of our Lord recorded exclusively in Luke's gospel: "Likewise even as it came to pass in the days of Lot; they ate, they drank, they bought, they sold, they planted, they builded; but in the day that Lot went out from Sodom it rained fire and brimstone from heaven, and destroyed them all: after the same manner shall it be in the day that the Son of man is revealed" (17:28–30, ASV). In regard to this matter of eating, drinking, buying, selling, planting and building, there is nothing here that is not normal for mankind, nothing in itself of a sinful nature, nothing which would warrant the terrible destruction of Sodom and Gomorrah. We must turn back to the book of Genesis, to the description of those conditions of these cities of the plain, that led to this divine destruction. It was nothing else but homosexuality,

normally called until recent times by a much uglier word deriving from Sodom's name.

Within two years of the Stonewall riots, homosexual visibility had become a serious concern for Christian fundamentalists.[4]

During the 1970s, probably the best known American evangelical Christian was David Wilkerson, author of a book immensely popular among born-again Protestants, *The Cross and the Switchblade*. According to David Edwin Harrell, "no man's voice carried more authority in the charismatic revival" than Wilkerson. In a 1974 book, Wilkerson narrated a detailed vision of five calamities that he claimed to have received from God. Wilkerson prophesied:

> The sin of Sodom will again be repeated in our generation. Of all the sins Sodom was guilty of, the most grievous of all were the homosexual attacks by angry Sodomite mobs attempting to molest innocent people. Mass murderers have become commonplace in our generation. We witnessed the television news coverage of the Olympic massacre. Mass murder sprees have become so frequent that they are now almost taken for granted. The world is no longer shocked by these tragedies as in the past. The Bible says: "As it was in the days of Lot, so shall it also be in the days of the coming of the Son of Man." I have seen things in my vision which make me fear for the future of our children. I speak of wild, roving mobs of homosexual men publicly assaulting innocent people in parks, on the streets, and in secret places. These attacks by Sodomite mobs are certain to come, and, although they may not be publicized as such, those in the law-enforcement circles will know the full extent of what is happening.

Wilkerson engaged a conspiratorial paranoia that alleged the certainty of these events, even though they may occur "in secret places" and "may not be publicized as such." This free associated "vision" remarkably elided sodomy with murder, a linkage Wilkerson made even more explicitly in his section entitled, "A Homosexual Epidemic":

> There are only two forces that hold back homosexuals from giving themselves over completely to their sin, and they are rejection by society and the repudiation and teachings of the church. When society no longer rejects their sin as abnormal and fully accepts them and encourages them in their abnormality, and when the church no longer preaches

against it as sin and consoles them in their sexual activities—there no longer exist any hindering forces. The floodgates are open, and homosexuals are encouraged to continue in their sin. In my vision, I have seen these two roadblocks being swept away. When that which hinders is taken away, chaos will follow. Believe me when I tell you the time is not far off that you will pick up your local newspaper and read sordid accounts of innocent children being attacked by wild homosexual mobs in parks and on city streets. The mass rapes will come just as surely as predicted in the Gospels. I see them coming in our generation. Twenty-seven boys were murdered in Houston, Texas, by a small homosexual gang. This sordid news story is the beginning of many other such tragic outbreaks. You can expect more than one homosexual scandal in very high places. The homosexual community will become so militant and brazen that they will flaunt their sin on television talk shows very shortly. Very clearly, I see homosexuals coming out in mass numbers and deviate sex crimes becoming more numerous and vicious.

Of course, since then, much more has been flaunted on television talk shows than militant and brazen homosexuality, most of it having to do with heterosexual eroticism, and where precisely in the gospels a prophecy of such events can be found is not clear. Wilkerson's rhetorical demonizing alloyed sensationalist references to news events with parental anxieties about their children's safety and the white middle class's apprehensions about rioting mobs; the admixture was effective in creating a sense of urgency and terror. It was a remarkable blend of biblical proof texts with supermarket tabloid rhetoric.[5]

Wilkerson was not the first religious writer to equate homosexuality with epidemic disease, nor was he the last. One widely published and popular evangelical fundamentalist, Tim LaHaye, wrote in 1978 that "America is experiencing a homosexual epidemic" and interpreted Israelite history to contend that the Babylonian captivity was in part the result of homosexuality. He claimed that "many Bible scholars think one of the major sins that brought on the Flood was homosexuality" and offered a fairly detailed historiographic inventory of homosexually-decadent societies including Pompeii, Rome, Athens, and post-World War II Britain. LaHaye was explicit in his apocalyptic reading of homosexuality: "Most Bible prophecy scholars teach that we are either in 'the last days,' predicted in the Scriptures, or we are very close to them. Interestingly enough, homosexuality is to be a part of the buildup of the 'perilously evil times' that are prophesied for the last days."[6]

Similarly, in *Power in the Blood: A Christian Response to AIDS*, David Chilton quoted Rousas John Rushdoony's 1973 *The Institutes of Biblical Law*: "Homosexuality is thus the culminating sexual practice of a culminating apostasy and hostility towards God. The homosexual is at war with God, and, in his every practice, is denying God's natural order and law. The theological aspect of homosexuality is thus emphasized in Scripture. In history, homosexuality becomes prominent in every age of apostasy and time of decline. It is an end of an age phenomenon." Another early fundamentalist tract on homosexuality, David A. Noebel's *The Homosexual Revolution: A Look at the Preachers and Politicians Behind It*, cited both biblical and historiographic authority:

> Scripture makes it exceeding clear that homosexuality is a mark of social decline. History records that the Greek, Roman, Persian and Moslem civilizations declined as homosexuality became more prevalent within those cultures. Homosexuals have a tendency to turn against their parent society if it does not succumb to homosexuality. They will subvert their own nation if they consider it to be too moral or anti-homosexual. The American public must make its decision: Will America maintain a Biblical valued system and move toward moral health and restoration, or will She follow other civilizations on the road to paganism and decay?

Here again, the historical moment was presented as a crisis in the terms of two irreconcilable opposites.[7] A California Congressman, William Dannemeyer, writing later in the decade, would repeat the historiographic claim that:

> [I]n the greatest of civilizations, there is usually a common thread at the end, a corruption of spirit that leads to selfishness and preoccupations with pleasure, eventually to the exclusion of what is usual and normal. At that point, excess and perversion come into fashion, and after that—catastrophe. There are numerous examples of such decadence, and at the end of great civilizations you almost always find homosexuality—widespread, energetic, enormously proud of itself.

He also offered Rome, the Mayan civilization, Venice, and Weimar Germany as exemplars of homosexually-induced decline.[8]

After the scandal-driven collapse of Bryant's Protect America's Children and Anita Bryant Ministries, her executive director wrote in 1984:

> The road to ruin for America has been paved by the political homo-
> sexual militants. Their program is conceived in wickedness. Their plat-
> form is morally perverse. They would lead America to disaster, just as
> their ancient counterparts led Sodom to its certain doom.

America was typologically configured as both Sodom and ancient Greece,
and homosexuality or even only tolerance of homosexuality leads it along
the "road to ruin," thus simultaneously constructing a crisis and demonizing homosexuals. Rowe read homosexual behavior—even the social
tolerance of homosexual behavior—as not simply a harbinger of the end
times but even as the cause of such an apocalyptic rupture in American
history. Beyond this historical exegesis, what makes Rowe's account even
more interesting than Bryant's, is its further demonization of homosexuals as "anti-God, anti-Christ, anti-Bible, anti-moral, anti-life, anti-
constitutional and anti-American."[9]

Apocalyptic Discourse

The readiness of HIV/AIDS affected/infected culture workers to employ
a religious discourse typically associated with groups who stigmatized
both AIDS and the earliest visible victims of the syndrome, gay men,
indicates some of the resilience of this ancient discursive form as well
as its pervasiveness in American cultural life. The "slipperiness" of
apocalypticism—its ability to serve competing ideologies—may be produced by the polysemous character of religious discourse generally. Pierre
Bourdieu in *Language and Symbolic Power* claimed that "The polysemy of
religious language, and the ideological effect of the *unification of opposites*
or denial of divisions which it produces, derive from the fact that, at the
cost of the *re-interpretations* implied in the production and reception of the
common language by speakers occupying different positions in the social
space, and therefore endowed with different intentions and interests, it
manages to speak to all groups and all groups speak it." Robert Hodge
might agree without making special claims for religious language:

> [S]imilar forms can be used by non-dominant groups as strategies of
> resistance, which are no more (and no less) compromised by this simi-
> larity than is the case with ideological complexes in the discourse of the
> dominant. . . . [W]e clearly cannot assume a single automatic value of

'dominant' or 'resistant' for any ideological form. Instead we need to accept contradiction and instability as the typical features of ideology as it appears in discourse, in criticism and in literature.[10]

The master's tools might not disassemble the master's house, but see what work can be done with them! Apocalyptic discourse is particularly effective in promoting group solidarity by engaging the individual and collective sense of threat and crisis. Early in the epidemic, AIDS was a crisis for those immediately affected by it as well as those who simply viewed its spectacle. The apocalypse is equally at home at the service of radicals and reactionaries.

Apocalypticism, according to Barry Brumett, has "undergirded Western thought for centuries, embodied in such central secular ideas as progress, manifest destiny, economic growth, and scientific advance" as well as in the obvious religious contexts. M. H. Abrams alternatively argues that the resilience of this form in Western culture may result in part from the pervasiveness of the Bible in the production of Western texts. Similarly, Brummett points out that "[a]pocalyptic is not the *only* way to deal with looming disorder, but it is a venerable and important one." Millennialism, the belief in the possibility of a perfect society either through a benign divinity (the faith of Christianity) or benign economic and historical forces (the faith of both Marxism and capitalism), and the revolutions necessary to produce such utopian conditions have been attributed to apocalyptic ideologies. However, I would caution against reading apocalyptic discourse only for revolutionary or protorevolutionary ideologies since millennialism can also be used to support the established order in crisis, which according to Ernest R. Sandeen, is apparently at work in the regressive politics of Christian fundamentalism and implicit in fundamentalism's apocalyptic roots.[11]

In particular, I am interested in how apocalyptic discourse constructs the "identity" and cohesiveness of a community under stress in such a way that a group has one instrument to negotiate with the volatility of a crisis. I see apocalyptic discourse constructing this identity in two related ways: by deploying a series of binary oppositions, which proceed from Self/Other, and by employing anxieties about physical defilement as one means of enforcing the binary oppositions. The binaristic character of apocalyptic discourse has been widely noted. Paul Ricouer suggested that this dualistic character derives first from mythic notions of theogonic combat, in which the world is created by a battle; with the introduction of the Hebrew Genesis myth of benign origins, this combat is transposed into the historical realm (i.e., the king and his enemies). Charles Lippy proposes that:

> apocalyptic groups emerge with tight boundaries, and a strong sense of their corporate identity and distinctiveness, a view of the universe as a battleground between forces of good and evil (with evil momentarily holding the upper hand), and an intense concern to protect pure believers from constant attack by polluting forces.[12]

The construction of identity by means of a series of binary oppositions (e.g., Self/Other, Us/Them, sacred/secular) is then reinforced by the representation of physical defilement.

Apocalyptic texts frequently betray a preoccupation with physical purity and a concomitant anxiety about physical defilement, including defiling excrements and disgusting smells. Couliano observes that "Zoroastrianism translates this entire series of binary oppositions into olfactory terms, that is, fragrant as opposed to foul." Furthermore, he notes "how frequently crimes derive from pollution and to what extent punishment is olfactory." In constructing the Self by means of demonizing the Other, apocalyptic discourse relishes almost obsessively the forms of defilement leading to punishments that consist of further physical defilement:

> The main sins seem to be sexual, but not all are. Thus, we find in hell Sodomites; women who touched water and fire while menstruating; men who copulated with women during their menstrual period; adulterous women; people who urinated while standing; . . . people who did not take a ritual bath after polluting water and fire . . . Most of these unfortunate inmates of hell, in fact, gorge themselves with excrement . . . elsewhere we find women hung upside down, with 'the semen of all kinds of demons,' stench, and filth poured continuously into their mouths and noses, for having denied their husbands intercourse.

In the *Apocalypse of Peter*, an apocryphal second-century Christian text, mothers who killed their children have a ceaseless flow of milk from their breasts that "congeals and smells foul, and from it come forth beasts that devour flesh, which turn and torture them for ever." Usurers find themselves in a "great lake, full of discharge and blood and boiling mire." The "discharge and the excrement of the tortured" runs down to form a lake, where women who had children out of wedlock are consigned. The fourth-century *Apocalypse of Paul* describes in detail the stench of the well of the abyss to which heretics are consigned.[13]

Not only the ancient texts but later medieval and early modern apocalyptic discourses achieved a voyeuristic obsession with the details of infernal punishments that bordered on the pornographic, as Bernard Capp suggested in the case of one early English Protestant:

> The symbol of evil, seductive Whore of Babylon (Rev. xvii) sometimes stirred darker, subconscious passions. They are all too clear, for example in Thomas Brightman's wish to "see this impudent harlot at length slit in the nostrils, stripped of her garments and tires [attire], besmearched with dirt and rotten eggs, and at last burnt up and consumed with fire."

Ricouer noted that the "inflation of the sexual is characteristic of the whole system of defilement, so that an indissoluble complicity between sexuality and defilement seems to have been formed from time immemorial." It is as though all sexuality is defiling, but some must be sanctioned or permitted, albeit controlled:

> Do not the marriage rites, among others, aim to remove the universal impurity of sexuality by marking out an enclosure within which sexuality ceases to be a defilement, but threatens to become so again if the rules concerning times, places, and sexual behavior are not observed?

Ricouer pointed out the association of sexuality with contamination, and the archaic linking of vengeance with defilement, so that defilement produces dread. Dread of vengeance for a "violated interdict" sees suffering as a symptom or product of sin, providing the typical theodicy of both prophetic and apocalyptic discourse. This theodicy ("Bad things happen to bad people") is predominant in the Judaeo-Christian tradition, though only paradoxically so, since the scriptural traditions of both Christians and Jews explicitly acknowledge that sometimes bad things happen to good people. And the notion that tribulations will touch the faithful is a staple of American apocalypticism as far back as the New England Puritans.[14] The identity of the social collective or of the individual within that collective is jeopardized by the blurring or transgression of boundaries, which are for the most part arbitrary. Thus in the irreducible logic of the economy of defilement, heretics are sexual "deviates," sexual "deviates" are heretics, and so both must ingest excreta; painting the demonic Other requires a broad (often excrement-soaked) brush.

Julia Kristeva made this point in *Powers of Horror: An Essay on Abjection*: "It is thus not lack of cleanliness or health that causes abjection but what disturbs identity, system, order. What does not respect borders, positions, rules. The in-between, the ambiguous, the composite." The defilement of body materials like urine, blood, sperm, excrement "collapse the border between inside and outside" but are simultaneously repulsive and fascinating. Social collectives, in her view, manage defilement by a series of rituals and taboos in order to construct collective identity, negotiating between sublimation and perversion at their crossing in religious practice. In particular for an understanding of the binary operation of apocalyptic discourse, Kristeva offers the interesting observation that Christian apocalypticism shares with earlier Semitic traditions "[a]n identical sacred horror for the feminine, the diabolical, and the sexual . . . by means of an incantation whose particular prosody confirms the name of the genre: a discovering, a baring of truth." Kristeva generalizes on this notion when she asserts:

> On close inspection, all literature is probably a version of the apocalypse that seems to me rooted, no matter what its socio-historical conditions might be, on the fragile border (borderline cases) where identities (subject/object, etc.) do not exist or only barely so—double, fuzzy, heterogeneous, animal, metamorphosed, altered, abject.[15]

This phenomenology applied to the apocalyptic discourses of AIDS, I would argue, represents a psychosocial dynamic that was at work throughout the 1970s in the increasing visibility and articulation of homosexual desires and homosexual bodies, prompting some people to repulse or abject violently these homosexual signs. American Christian fundamentalists felt imperiled by the convulsive social changes in the 1960s and 1970s, especially around issues of gender and sexuality. Even before the "epiphany" of AIDS, religious conservatives had already employed lurid images of homosexual defilement and the binary oppositions of apocalyptic discourse. Both configurations intensified with the gradually wider public awareness of the medical syndrome around 1983 precisely because discussions of its transmission had to take into account the remarkably diverse range of human sexual behaviors, which included public discourse about body fluids and products, traditionally defiling substances.

Because this book examines how HIV/AIDS affected/infected culture workers in New York City appropriated apocalyptic tropes in an effort to resist or reverse them, I need to provide an account of this discourse and its associated ideologies in a particular and concrete historical situation. To do so I will employ a critical method that accounts for genre, form, and the concrete social and historical givens of specific texts, a critical method that allows for useful generalizations without losing the particularities. In what follows, I will briefly summarize some of the more incisive critiques of AIDS apocalypticism and explain the social semiotic analysis that will provide the critical tools for this study.

AIDS, APOCALYPTICISM, AND CULTURE CRITICISM

Culture workers of HIV/AIDS affected/infected communities appropriated apocalyptic tropes in their own resistive discourse. From mainstream authors to activists and biomedical journalists to performance artists, this cultural production employed various apocalyptic commonplaces: universal destruction, beastly and demonic evil, conspiracy theories, tropes of plague and pestilence, images of blood and defilement, jeremiadic and oracular utterances, narratives of otherworldly journeys and messengers, and fantasies of utopic or paradisal reunion. However, not all culture analysts found this apocalyptic rhetoric appropriate or useful in the struggle for advocacy on behalf of those living with AIDS.

By the early 1990s queer apocalyptic representations of AIDS were ubiquitous, and the facility with which gay men in particular adopted an apocalyptic stance to manage the implications of the epidemic was not without its critics. Gay writer and activist Darrel Yates Rist's antiapocalyptic 1989 article, "AIDS as Apocalypse: The Deadly Costs of an Obsession," pointed out that "[T]his panicky faith that all of us are doomed cries down the sobering truth that it is only a minority of homosexuals who've been stricken or ever will be, leaving the rest of us to confront not so much the grief of dying as the bitterness, in an oppressive world, of staying alive."[16] Rist suggested that the rhetoric was counterproductive and more than a little dishonest. Similarly, in *AIDS and Its Metaphors* Susan Sontag pointed out the postmodern paradox of the intensification of apocalyptic rhetoric contrasted with the simultaneous deferral of an actual apocalyptic rupture. This premillennialism is symptomatic of the postmodern condition: "Apocalypse is now a long-running serial: not 'Apocalypse Now' but 'Apocalypse from Now On,' " a postmodernity particularly typical of American culture. Analogously, she associated this apocalypticism with "an end-of-an-era feeling" prevalent in our culture and intensified by AIDS. Both apocalyptic discourse and fin de siècle style are homologous of catastrophe and only catastrophe: "That even an apocalypse can be made to seem part of the ordinary horizon of expectation constitutes an unparalleled violence that is being done to our sense of reality, to our humanity." However, Sontag's analysis on this point is weakened because she employed "apocalypse" only in its most limited (though popular) sense of cataclysm; thus she failed to see its recuperative possibilities. She also confused entropic fin de siècle style with utopic apocalypticism, blending post-Romanticism with Judaeo-Christian eschatology, seeming to elide significant differences between European and American discourses and cultures.[17]

Other culture critics were inclined, like Rist and Sontag, to interrogate the apocalyptic significations of AIDS. James Miller remarked that "Without faith to limit apocalyptic fantasy, hell hardly differs from history as constructed on the nightly news." He proposed the "anastatic moment . . . the illuminative climax of the personal or public struggles of the bereaved to make sense of death" as a critical term to understand what is going on in many representations of AIDS. For Miller, the anastatic moment is a kind of resurrection (without explicit religious faith) and he examined the reinvention of heaven in several AIDS elegies in which Fire Island is figured as Paradise. Miller's article was dedicated to the memory of Michael Lynch, fellow Canadian and AIDS activist who died in 1991. Too debilitated with AIDS-related illness to present a paper at the 1988 Modern Language Association Convention, Lynch instructed that his paper, entitled "Terrors of Resurrection 'by Eve Kosofsky Sedgwick' " be presented *in absentia* by Sedgwick, his Duke University colleague. Lynch argued the need for alternatives to apocalyptic discourse in AIDS writing, which are problematic because of "[T]heir distance from lives as led." He suggested that there is even some resistance to viewing AIDS as anything but apocalyptic, a resistance to viewing HIV infection as simply another (manageable) disease (the article was written during the hopeful introduction of one of the first HIV drugs, AZT). The challenge for Lynch was viewing AIDS "[N]ot as apocalypse now, nor as apocalyptic from now on, but as getting the FDA and the NIH to expedite treatments, as working out manageable workloads with employers or thesis supervisors, as figuring out ways to cope with recurrent nausea, as figuring out ways to get down a *whole* peanut butter sandwich, as making time, not serving it." Lynch resisted producing a cosmic meaning around HIV infection and AIDS, and viewed the syndrome instead as a medical management issue. Peter Dickinson's ""Go-go Dancing on the Brink of the Apocalypse': Representing AIDS" offered a critique of "abstract theorizing about AIDS," suggested that neither AIDS nor apocalypticism exists outside of the discursive practices that represent it, and performed a "taxonomy of the various modes of apocalypse at work in the discursive production of AIDS—from the marketing of apocalypse by biomedicine and the media to the ironizing of apocalypse by gay activists and artists—paying particular attention to the representation of identity and difference, safer sex, and persons living with AIDS and HIV." In each instance, culture critics have noticed that both the political right (whom one might expect to employ biblical tropes) and the political left (whom one might be surprised to find using scriptural figures) have employed apocalyptic discourses, but have done so at a price to the people living under the threat of AIDS.[18]

Feminist critics have also applied their own interventions to apocalyptic discourses, observing the ways in which those discourses are typically scripted around sexual-defilement and gender anxieties. Their attitudes toward apocalypticism, however, are quite varied. Catherine Keller's theological *Apocalypse Now and Then* suggests that one can "remain accountable . . . to the cultural hunger for a spirituality that might actually compete with apocalyptic fundamentalisms on behalf of sustainable and shared life in the present. This means at least taking the biblical text seriously." Her project is to recuperate the liberatory possibilities of apocalypticism for marginalized people. She does not imagine an end of endism, an apocalypse of apocalypticism, but hopes instead to revise the text. By contrast, in *Apocalyptic Bodies: The Biblical End of the World in Text and Image*, Tina Pippin attempts to resist rather than revise these texts. She is fascinated and repulsed by the Book of Revelation's treatment of women's bodies, but also fascinated by its queerly ambiguous treatment of men's bodies. However, she concludes that its "message is still not liberating for our late twentieth-century feminist and pro-gay liberation movements. Of course, I am using twentieth-century language and terms to define a first-century world view. I make this hermeneutical leap because I want to figure out how to read the Apocalypse in this century of genocide and Aids."[19] Similarly, in two concise and carefully argued texts, *Anti-Apocalypse: Exercises in Genealogical Criticism* and *Millennial Seduction: A Skeptic Confronts Apocalyptic Culture*, Lee Quinby employs a feminist commitment with Foucauldian analysis. In *Anti-Apocalypse*, she observes the dual possibilities of apocalypticism: mobilization or passivity. Like Tina Pippin she regards apocalyptic discourses with suspicion and her goals in this earlier book are to analyze and resist the antidemocratic tendencies that she views as intrinsic to these discourses. Unlike Keller, however, Quinby imagines an end of endism, the apocalypse of apocalypticism. In what she characterizes as "pissed criticism" she examines the apocalyptic anxieties of physical/sexual defilement that coalesced about AIDS and "bodily fluids." Her later book, *Millennial Seductions*, offers Tony Kushner's *Angels in America* as a paradigm for moral education, with its "threshold of revelation" challenging "both the fatalistic view that nothing can be done to change the world and the relativistic view that the moral standing of a given act depends on the moral belief of the actor, regardless of consequences to others." Quinby advances her antiapocalypticism as an antidote to apocalypticism's antidemocratic script, which in recent years the Religious Right has employed against gender and sexual pluralism.[20]

The most extensive critical treatment of AIDS and apocalypticism is Richard Dellamora's *Apocalyptic Overtures: Sexual Politics and the Sense of an Ending*. Dellamora argues that

> [T]he association of sex between men with end times is embedded in the political unconscious of Christian societies. Accordingly, when persecution of such subjects increases at moments, such as the ends of centuries, when cultural anxieties about time become intensified, such responses are due not only to immediate but also to atavistic factors.

The instances of this conjunction and the fact that both dominant groups and subordinate groups employ apocalyptic discourse for their own purposes lead Dellamora to express caution in their reading and to invoke both Derrida and Foucault. Deconstruction for Dellamora is both a site of apocalyptic theory and its critique; in the West, philosophy "[A]lways occurs within an apocalyptic metadiscourse" about the "ends of man" that is often universalized, while Derridean deconstruction offers both an analytic and an affirmative moment: "The first is necessary in order to resist the manipulative use of apocalyptic discourse. The second is necessary in order to mobilize the discourse on behalf of subordinated individuals and groups." Foucault offers a similarly binary "tactical productivity" and "strategical integration" as terms of the analysis of discourse.[21]

These analytical tools acknowledge both the democratic and the totalitarian possibilities of apocalypticism. Dellamora applies them to nineteenth-century fin de siècle sensibility, twentieth-century gay/queer writing, and representations of AIDS or AIDS-era writing, the last including Neil Bartlett's 1988 novel *Who Was That Man? A Present for Mr Oscar Wilde*, Edmund White's 1986 short story, "An Oracle," and Andrew Hollinghurst's 1988 novel invoking a pre-AIDS past, *The Swimming Pool Library*.[22] More than any other critic, Dellamora recognizes both the utopic and the entropic possibilities in apocalyptic discourse, and emphasizes the pervasiveness of this discourse in American social and political life. His analysis makes explicit in a way no other critic has done the coincidence of Western apocalyptic narrative and homosexual anxieties.

At the same time, however, Dellamora constructs his analysis upon texts that seem to me atypical of American writing: British or European for the most part, rather than North American—Bartlett, Wilde, Pater, Hollinghurst, the early Burroughs, the part-time expatriate White. And Derridean deconstruction, all protests to the contrary notwithstanding, dehistoricizes texts and reads them for what they "might do" rather than for what they "have done." Deconstruction in this case does not provide an adequately pragmatic analysis of AIDS and apocalypticism. To me, Dellamora's most satisfying chapter is the three-page "Afterword," where he recounts attending a performance of David Drake's *The Night Larry Kramer Kissed Me* and where Dellamora defines the effects that the play—and its concluding apocalyptic turn—produced upon him and other audience members, while he contextualizes the play in its material performance space: a nineteenth-century West Village police stable, converted into a theater a few years after Stonewall, and later renovated and dedicated to queer theater in 1988. His account at that point engages a world outside of the text—or a world, perhaps, in which the text is enlarged—where texts are more than verbal and are written on bodies and buildings as much as in books. It is precisely such an examination of the material effects of discourses on real bodies that interests me here, and for this reason I propose that a historicist social semiotics might make a valuable contribution to the critical analysis of AIDS discourses that has been advanced thus far.[23]

SOCIAL SEMIOTICS

Making a claim for a formal identity over time and across cultures among texts employing similar discursive structures and conventions, requires a theoretical account of an apocalyptic genre, while at the same time an effective praxis demands an account that is not reductively formalistic or dehistoricized. Although there is no essential "form" of apocalypse, and although no monolithic or univocal definition of the term has successfully prevailed in scholarly discourse, there is a widely accepted sense of "family resemblances" that construct the apocalyptic genre. Attention to points of resemblance, however, can lead to a formalistic and taxonomic analysis of texts and performances that reduces difference and evades their material historic contingencies. Social semiotics is one critical tool that evades formalism, while accounting for the conventions that constitute genre, by attending to the historical materiality of texts and performances and by acknowledging that "style" is an ideological construction rather than the object of aesthetic contemplation. Social semiotics can also be applied to a range of discursive practices (verbal texts, performance, iconic visual arts) because all discourses are viewed as situated on the larger landscape of the social production of meaning, while their contradictions are understood as inherent in social negotiations of identity and power, solidarity and exclusion.[24] This study, for example, will examine not only "literary" texts and other verbal (including journalistic and biomedical) texts, but also performance art, films, ACT-UP demonstrations and graphics, and other visual arts in an attempt to assess the tactical and strategic instrumentality of apocalyptic discourse in particular cases.

At the base of a semiotic analysis is the recognition that

> [T]exts are both the material realization of systems of signs, and also the site where change continually takes place. The dialectic between text and system always occurs in specific semiosic acts, that is, in discourse. Discourse in this sense is the site where social forms of organization engage with systems of signs in the production of texts, thus reproducing or changing the sets of meanings and values which make up a culture.[25]

In the continuous exchanges between dominant groups and dominated groups there occurs affirmation of, accommodation of and resistance to values, meanings, and behaviors. (The seemingly facile dichotomizing of the social site into "dominant" and "dominated" belies the complex subjectivity of postmodern urban life, in which individuals might inhabit simultaneously several dominant and dominated subject positions, while perceiving themselves as inhabiting still others.) Both Christian fundamentalists and the HIV/AIDS affected/infected will have understood themselves as "dominated" by a destructive hegemony that threatens their very existence, and in this study I will explore how the latter group has employed apocalyptic discourse derived not only from the immediate discursive field of American sexual politics in the late 1970s and early 1980s, but also from a more extensive cultural pattern in American society.

In the first decade of the AIDS epidemic this contestatory site and its competing ideologies produced "ideological complexes," that is to say "a functionally related set of contradictory versions of the world, coercively imposed by one social group on another on behalf of its own distinctive interests or subversively offered by another social group in attempts at resistance in its own interests,"[26] operating within the set of rules called a "logonomic system." Logonomic systems establish identity and solidarity and enforce power by controlling the production of meaning:

> [W]ho can think and say what to whom in what way, and who or what is excluded from discourse and knowledge. This control is exercised by rules, implicit or explicit, concerning the major elements of the semiosic process: producers and receivers, texts and topics. Rules concerned with these can be termed *production regimes, reception regimes, genre regimes,* and *noetic regimes* respectively.[27]

Apocalyptic discourse (like all discourse but more ostentatiously so, perhaps) produces social identity, cohesion, and coherence by its construction of subjects and objects (or often, abjects). However, despite the implication of "control . . . by rules" the semiotic process is not mechanistically determined; therefore "[s]ocial semiotics cannot assume that texts produce exactly the meanings and effects that their authors hope for: it is precisely the struggles and their uncertain outcomes that must be studied at the level of social action, and their effects in the production of meaning."[28]

One task of this study will be to interrogate specific cultural productions in a specific place and time in order to determine the effects of social action. Within logonomic systems, genre regimes covertly engage production and reception and noetic regimes by adjudicating, not simply the classification of existing texts, but behavior and thought, how authors write and readers interpret, what they should write and read about; thus genre regimes classify more than existing texts but also classify people— "readers and writers—and . . . what they write or read about and what they should think and mean," producing both ideology and identity. Apocalypticism has a cultural history as a genre, a genealogy that is not accidental to its ideological freight and social effects, nowhere more so than in its American configurations.[29]

Material texts (and performances similarly) do not exist in isolation but are situated in a context or domain, that is "categories of place associated with kinds of meaning and kinds of semiosic agent."[30] Thus *domain* will become a useful critical category of this study in two ways: examining the transformation of apocalyptic tropes from an explicitly Christian religious domain to a variety of secularized domains; and examining differences among those secularized domains (as, for example, in the second chapter's critique of a novel about a performance artist; a high-profile, nationally known off-Broadway performance piece; and an "alternative" performance piece).[31] Similarly, the analysis of textual style, rather than an object of the formalist's gaze, is a critique of ideology, since

> The more distinctive (different, marked) the style of a text or genre, the more strongly the existence of an anti-group is signaled, conscious of its opposition to other groups in society, so that high stylization is a transparent signifier of high polarization and conflict. And secondly, the meanings coded in form and style will be core meanings in dispute that organize group against group, so that this class of meanings is indispensable to a comprehensive analysis of intellectual movements in a social history of thought.[32]

The significance of apocalyptic "style" is fundamentally concerned with group identity and solidarity, the construction of authorized "authors" and initiated "readers," partly through its extreme and allegorical tropes.[33]

AMERICAN APOCALYPTICISM

Apocalypticism is one possible response to threats to group identity and cohesion. That apocalyptic discourse should typify some Americans' response to epidemic disease is not surprising given its pervasiveness throughout American history. Numerous critics and historians have argued that apocalypticism was a founding motive and a foundational discourse of the Spanish and English settlement of the Americas and particularly of the New England colonies, which was continued through their cultural and intellectual dominance up until the early twentieth century.[34] When

Americans resort to defining social turning points in terms of catastrophic crisis, we are engaging in apocalyptic discourse. When we redefine our commitments to social action by declaring metaphorical (and sometimes literal) *war*, as for example the War on Poverty, the War on Drugs, the War on Terrorism, even the War to End All Wars, we are engaging in apocalyptic discourse. When we define social and political boundaries in binary *oppositions*, inevitably naming a demon or hunting a witch, we are engaging in apocalyptic discourse. When we construct our past and fantasize our future in terms of a prophetic and utopic *mission*, we are engaging in apocalyptic discourse. One does not need to believe in a religion or its prophecies to reproduce the language of apocalypticism. This mode of constructing meaning has become naturalized in our national language. Seventeenth-century Puritan apocalypticism has a remarkably long half-life, continuing to radiate most American discourse as we begin the twenty-first century.[35]

Composing an American apocalyptic genealogy fulfills two functions: to identify the ideological and discursive headwaters of today's millennialism and to suggest affinities between past and current deployment of those fluid beliefs and languages, in particular the conflation of apocalyptic desires, sexual anxieties, and contagion. One might trace such ancestors beginning with the first European colonization of the Americas. In part Christopher Columbus' prophetic pretensions impelled his westward exploration on behalf of Spanish monarchs who had only recently expelled the last Moorish infidels and Jews from their kingdom.[36] Jonathan Goldberg has ably described the antisodomitical violence of both the Spanish and English colonizers in the Americas, who conflated racial difference with sexual and religious difference, rendering the native Other as both sodomitical and heretical.[37]

To his discussion I would graft an understanding of the characteristically *apocalyptic vehemence* that energizes colonial antisodomitical violence, especially in the New English colonies.[38] Earnest Cassara argues that the New England Puritans exercised a cultural dominance that persists in some vestiges today, particularly in many Americans' belief in their divinely ordained mission. Cassara points out that Puritan "[i]ntolerance was part of their contract with God. They had moved across the ocean to erect in New England the English church in purified form. To maintain that purity in the face of both internal and external threats, intolerance became state policy." Tuveson makes the same point when he characterizes Christian apocalypticism as possessing a dualism with no room for middle ground, a belief in tribulation prior to victory, in condoning purging violence, and in a progressive view of history, as well as in manifest destiny, as the nineteenth century would phrase it. Moreover, the Puritans tended to view keeping the community free of defilement not simply as an ethical ideal, but as an existential necessity: a question of survival or doom. As Kathleen Verduin observes: "Reinforcing a world view essentially punitive in nature, New England ministers like Danforth and the Mathers linked sexuality with deeper, indeed fundamental, threats: atheism, paganism, and apocalyptic judgment."[39]

American apocalyptic expectations were quickened from the time of Cotton Mather, Jonathan Edwards, and the Great Awakening earlier in the eighteenth century toward the time of the Revolutionary War. Robert Fuller suggests that many colonists would have identified the Antichrist with the Church of Rome and in particular its French surrogates in North America; but after the French and Indian War, the British king himself came to be characterized as the beast. As Lakshmi Mani observes, "During the Revolutionary era, the American Revolution came to be hailed on both sides of the Atlantic as the millennium," a phenomenon Henry F. May characterized as a "Secular Millennialism." According to J. F. Maclear numerous apologists for the Revolution sought "to locate the new American nation in a grand apocalyptic interpretation of universal history, the only conceptual framework acceptable to a people still rooted in the providential assumptions of the English Reformation." By the time of the early republic, a literary as well as a religious apocalypticism was firmly in place.[40]

Epidemic disease represented in terms of apocalyptic panic is characteristic of one of the Early Republic's first novels: Charles Brockden Brown's *Arthur Mervyn*, published in 1799 and 1800 and based on the Philadelphia yellow fever epidemic of 1793. Philadelphia at the time was the new republic's seat of government and an economically and culturally significant capital as well.[41] As J. H. Powell has remarked in his history of the first epidemic, "The yellow fever, before the death of the young men whose first plague was 1793, became the most thoroughly written-about disease in medicine. . . . Philadelphia's great plague, the first of a long series, attracted all the writers of medical history. It attracted other writers, too, those who saw moral and humanistic values in the plague." Norman S. Grabo indicates that Brown began the novel about two years after the epidemic, which he had witnessed during that summer, in a series of sketches that appeared in the Philadelphia *Weekly Magazine*. Publication of these installments was interrupted by another outbreak of yellow fever, which claimed the life of *Weekly Magazine* editor, James Watters, and Brown was to fall victim to a milder form of the fever after fleeing to New York City. In the eleventh installment we get a glimpse of Brown's ideological purposes that would later be appropriated into the novel when "The Man describes to a group of friends an act of ruthless political terrorism that silently and dreadfully destroys its enemies in silence, terror, and dread—a social allegory of the yellow fever itself. Clearly, Brown is indicating his awareness that the epidemic is social and moral as well as physical."[42]

The novel falls roughly into two parts, both of them first-person narratives, first by a Dr. Stevens telling what Mervyn told him, and then by Mervyn himself. Mervyn has come to Philadelphia from the countryside in order to seek his fortune, but is almost immediately exploited and conned. The innocent Mervyn travels to the city where he undergoes trials and testing, comes near death before being rescued by Dr. Stevens, and finally prevails over evil and arrives at marriage.

A major binary opposition of the novel is that between rural and urban settings. Mervyn ponders the differences between the two:

> I mused upon the incidents related by Estwick, upon the exterminating nature of this pestilence, and on the horrors of which it was productive. I compared the experience of the last hours, with those pictures which my imagination had drawn in the retirements of *Malverton*. I wondered at the contrariety that exists between the scenes of the city and the country; and fostered with more zeal than ever, the resolution to avoid those seats of depravity and danger.[43]

The city is the place of vice and plague that eventually infects the countryside. Brown refers to the city variously as "seat of infection" (128), "theatre of disasters," and "theatre of pestilence" (132), emphasizing the spectacular aspects of epidemic disease. The city is also a place of shifting identities and loyalties, whereas the country is generally the site of stability and community. Brown also constructs an opposition between truth and lies or honesty and dishonesty. The rural innocent, Mervyn attempts to read the slippery signifiers of the city, to pin down the ambiguous codes of a person's character. Even the currency that becomes a significant plot device may be "queer," since there is doubt whether it is genuine or forged. What is worse, with the onset of the epidemic, ties of friendship and family are abandoned:

The usual occupations and amusements of life were at an end. Terror had exterminated all the sentiments of nature. Wives were deserted by husbands, and children by parents. Some had shut themselves in their houses, and debarred themselves from all communication with the rest of mankind. The consternation of others had destroyed their understanding, and their misguided steps hurried them into the midst of the danger which they had previously laboured to shun. Men were seized by this disease in the streets; passengers fled from them; entrance into their own dwellings was denied to them; they perished in the public ways. The chambers of disease were deserted, and the sick left to die of negligence. None could be found to remove the lifeless bodies. Their remains, suffered to decay by piece-meal, filled the air with deadly exhalation, and added tenfold to the devastation. (122–23)

The city is thus a place of both moral and medical contagion from which the pristinely innocent countryside must defend itself.

Brown and his contemporaries made a variety of attempts to explain the source of the fever and to construct a meaning for the society afflicted with it. While many blamed outsiders (French emigrés from the revolution, Caribbean immigrants), a consensus developed attributing a local source. Mathew Carey's contemporary account suggested that:

Luxury, the usual, and perhaps inevitable concomitant of prosperity, was gaining ground in a manner very alarming to those who considered how far the virtue, the liberty, and the happiness of a nation depend on its temperance and sober manners. . . . Not to enter into minute detail, let it suffice to remark, that extravagance, in various forms, was gradually eradicating the plain and wholesome habits of the city. And although it were presumption to attempt to scan the decrees of heaven, yet few, I believe, will pretend to deny, that something was wanting to humble the pride of a city, which was running on in full career, to the goal of prodigality and dissipation.

As John C. Miller pointed out in his study of the Alien and Sedition Acts, several years later *Greenleaf's New Daily Advertiser* would emphasize the depth of America's declension, blaming America's flirtation with French Jacobinism (as it saw it): "[W]e are a divided people, a degraded, insignificant, effeminate, dastardly race of beings, ready for the yoke." Alan Axelrod suggests that:

Arthur Mervyn . . . is a vision of the dis-ease of civilization in the New World. Brown, who had begun his literary career idly dreaming utopias, created in his most detailed portrait of an American city a plague-smitten, apocalyptic vision of an antiutopia, in which the only real sources of social relationship lie in a monetary system liable to counterfeiting and imposture or in sexual alliances smuggled into town as the counterfeiting fantasies of the asocial wilderness mind.

The contemporary apocalyptic construction of the yellow fever epidemic is apparent in Carey's account when he relates:

> Some of the Maryland papers relate, that 'a voice had been heard in the streets of Philadelphia, warning the inhabitants to prepare for their doom, as written in the prophet Ezekiel, ch. 27.' The Marylander who heard this voice, was certainly gifted with a most extraordinary ear, as, at the distance of above a hundred miles, he heard what we could not hear on the spot. And it would appear that his *sight* was equally good with his hearing; for he *saw* two angels conversing with the watch. It is true, he is too modest to say, he saw them himself—he only says 'two angels were *seen* conversing with the watch at midnight, about the subject of what the voice had previously proclaimed.'

Carey's ironic tone aside, contemporary accounts could read the epidemic as both punishment and warning.[44]

Yellow fever further destabilized the early republican government in a nation already imagining itself vulnerable to French Jacobinism, an anxiety eventually taking expression in the Alien and Sedition Laws. In June 1800 the *Gazette of the United States* proclaimed that, ""Our cities have been punished in proportion to the extent of Jacobinism; and in general at least three out of four of the person who have perished by pestilence have been over zealous partizans." As Shirley Samuels has pointed out, "the novel in this period reveals itself finally as a major locus for contemporary anxiety about the stability of the family and its freedom from unfaithfulness and the contamination of the outside world. Timothy Dwight, for example, configured Jacobin democracy [as] . . . a form of the yellow fever plague that had so terrorized Americans at the time of the Terror in France." In such a construction, ideology is contagious, and freedom of speech or freedom of representation is a threat to civic order, which is to say, civic identity. In colonial and early republican America, and today with remarkable continuity, our public discourse has coalesced around a ready-made repertoire of tropes of contamination and obliteration.[45]

The first fifteen years of AIDS representations showed a striking similarity to *Arthur Mervyn*'s "conflation of plague, politics, and sexual anxieties."[46] Numerous culture workers, activists, and others involved with AIDS appropriated this apocalyptic genealogy in New York City and other urban areas, between 1981 (the year of the disease's discursive epiphany) and 1996, the first decade and a half of the medical crisis. Since New York is both a prolific American cultural and discursive space, as well as an epicenter of the AIDS epidemic, it provides a rich venue for understanding the cultural production of meaning around this epidemic. But any focus entails two fictions that I must acknowledge now: a fiction of inclusion, in which items within the frame are perceived as contiguous and related, forming a "community"; and a fiction of exclusion, in which items outside the frame are relegated to silence and invisibility. Most of the instances of cultural production that I examine here are the work of gay white men, who had come to be so associated with AIDS precisely because of their discursive privilege relative to the cultural power of others affected by HIV/AIDS, a group that includes women, people of color, and drug users in significant numbers. In doing so, I am reflecting in part my own interests as a gay man affected by AIDS but also my access to this culture and its forms of cultural production. I will also try to resist representing New York's gay male population as a single, monolithic "gay community," an instrument of postmodern capitalism.[47] Just as the individual's subjectivity is continuously performed within a variety of often competing and sometimes conflicting subject positions, so social groups continuously redefine their boundaries and alliances. If in the late eighteenth century, public anxieties and uncriticized representations could result in repressive Alien and Sedition Laws, the same anxieties were the occasion in the late twentieth century's targeting of sexual dissidents. I also hope that this study will advance a therapeutic critique of one of America's more troublesome semiotic systems, apocalyptic discourse. In order to do so, I have organized this book around four apocalyptic tropes: exile as the crisis inciting the apocalyptic imagination; the prophetic jeremiad with its threats of doom; the final battle between good and evil, Armageddon; and ultimate paradisal bliss, configured in utopian and erotic terms.

In the next chapter, I will examine solo performance (perhaps the defining form of activist art in the late twentieth century) under the sign of exile (historically the disrupting catalyst for classic apocalyptic texts). Since World War II many queer people in "middle America" have experienced themselves as strangers in a strange land and Americans' response to AIDS only served to increase that alienation. Performers like David

Drake and Tim Miller explored that marginalization in their work, and, with an evangelical fervor, performed their solo pieces in order to counteract the stigmatizing and immobilizing effects of alienation. Similarly, a novella by an older generation writer, James McCourt, depicted a solo performance artist whose monologue is a kind of apocalypse, a book of revelation. In this chapter, I account for the material differences in the physical or psychic spaces in which these texts are performed (contrasting Drake's West Village venue, Miller's East Village and on-the-road venues, and McCourt's mainstream publication, or audiences for performances and readers of novels) as one way of understanding the effects they achieve. By discussing theorists like Judith Butler, David Román, Ed Cohen, Eve Kosofsky Sedgwick, and Peggy Phelan, I also test some of the (frequently inflated) claims made by performance theory in order to critique or qualify those claims.

The third chapter discusses the work of novelist and playwright Larry Kramer in light of a uniquely American discourse, the jeremiad. The American jeremiad turns on a contradiction: the imaginary cultural identity that posits a monolithic aristocracy of virtue (American exceptionalism) and the material reality of competing constituencies with conflicting values (American individualism), a contradiction whose ancestry extends to the first Puritan settlements in North America. The jeremiad, as Sacvan Bercovitch demonstrates, is effective only by means of "normalizing crisis," which eventually also proves to be its own undoing, since individuals and collectives can remain fixed for only so long (unless they are "true believers"). As a result, like most preachers of the jeremiad sermon, Kramer blazed into the public scene of AIDS activism attracting tremendous attention, but flickered out later, now largely ignored. Kramer's use of this discursive form predated his AIDS activism and it is found in his 1978 novel, *Faggots*.

Perhaps nothing so typifies American apocalypticism as our tendency to configure "normalized crises" in terms of war. Thus the fourth chapter examines the trope of Armageddon and the ease with which competing interests during the AIDS epidemic employed martial figures in order to mobilize a collective response. This chapter examines a variety of such instances—among AIDS organizations and militant (the word is advised) activists, ACT UP and its allied groups, Lesbian Avengers, right wing Christians—but pays particular attention to the fiction, journalism, and activism of Sarah Schulman. While the mobilizing efficacy of such rhetoric is undeniable, its usefulness comes at a price, namely by inscribing a fictional unity that erases important material differences among the constituencies working on behalf of AIDS treatment and prevention.

Finally, the end in classic apocalypses, the reward of the just, is imagined as a blissful union with divinity, a marriage of heaven and earth in the millennium. The fifth chapter examines tropes of sacred eros and millennialist ecstasy in two gay Jewish writers, Tony Kushner and Douglas Sadownick. Kushner and Sadownick both draw upon esoteric traditions—Jewish Kabbalah mysticism, Jungian alchemy, Neo-Platonism—that have antecedents in the early American Republic. Kushner's "great work," the epic plays that constitute *Angels in America*, perform what I call an "alchemy of symbolic capital" by their conjunction of disparate elements of American society in order to transmute them. If Kushner's luminous angel is descended from American transcendental Romanticism, Sadownick's leather "top" derives from our demonic or gothic Romanticism. In the novel *Sacred Lips of the Bronx* and in his nonfictional, obliquely Jungian *Sex Between Men: An Intimate History of the Sex Lives of Gay Men Postwar to Present*, Sadownick attempts to marry gay men's fragmented selves into wholeness. Thus Kushner is Whitman to Sadownick's Melville or Hawthorne. However, in both writers, the agenda is not simply a New Age narcissism, since their imaginations conceive an inclusive utopian politics.

Despite intellectuals' post-Enlightenment modernist tendency to view apocalyptic discourses as ranting from the fringes of society, those discourses are in fact central to the American experience and are quite effective in composing individual and collective identities by bestowing a coherence on fragmentary experience and by endowing the mundane with cosmic significance. The object of this study is to interrogate the ways in which disparate constituencies uncritically mobilize themselves through this *habitus*.

Chapter Two

Exile of the Queer Evangelist
(In memory of Michael)

This film scene is iconic for American popular culture generally and for gay culture, hypericonic: Miss Dorothy Gale of Kansas, having fled the black-and-white provincialism of her home, seeks a place where she and her companion are understood and accepted. She awakens to Technicolor, looks around her, and in a classic example of rhetorical litotes says to her little dog, "Toto, I don't think we're in Kansas anymore." In the years since its 1938 production, *The Wizard of Oz* has become a kind of sacred text for American gay culture largely because its structure and themes, turning on exile and quest, have spoken to the life situations of many queer people who likewise have sought a land of color and eccentricity in which they feel "normal" or "at home." In addition, the character of Dorothy Gale is enmeshed in the life of the actor portraying her, Judy Garland, whose gay icon status is legendary, so much so that her death and her wake at Frank Campbell's funeral home in New York are mythologically associated with the Stonewall riots in June 1969. Further, Garland's best known song from the film, "Somewhere Over the Rainbow," has become a kind of queer national anthem, and during the postwar regime of the closet, the phrase "friend of Dorothy" was a code to indicate one's queerness. A popular post-Stonewall postcard shows Dorothy anxiously clutching Toto in a leather bar saying, "Toto, I don't think we're in Kansas anymore."

Dorothy's cinematic exile and quest have represented for many late twentieth-century gay and lesbian people an image of their own search for identity and for a community where their desires might be honored and fulfilled. But no amount of ruby slippered heel clicking could return them to idyllic "homes" or families of birth. As many of those who developed AIDS discovered, their birth families were often as censorious about their dying as they were about their living: life-companions and friends excluded from medical and funeral arrangements or those too ill to take care of themselves remanded "home" or in some cases the dying simply abandoned by families of birth. Even today, queer folk often feel like exiles or "strangers in a strange land" among their blood kin and only feel at home when they have left their birth families to establish other households and families of affiliation.[1]

In this chapter I will explore exile as an apocalyptic sign, the trope of the speaking subject in crisis. In particular I will look at issues around performance and performativity, including the construction of space as a component of performance. Discourse about AIDS is imbricated with spatial figures, some of which I examine here in order to account for the material conditions of physical space. Finally, this chapter will discuss three pieces that represent "performance art": Tim Miller's *My Queer Body*, David Drake's *The Night Larry Kramer Kissed Me*, and James McCourt's *Time Remaining*. The first two, composed and performed by gay men in their twenties, are actual solo performance pieces, perhaps the defining genre of queer activist literature in the 1980s and 90s; the last, a stylistically complex novel written by a gay man in later midlife and published by a mainstream press. As I will show, those genre distinctions signify both different generational identities and material conditions.[2]

Stephen D. O'Leary reads apocalyptic texts as "dramatic enactment" with either tragic or comedic "frames of acceptance." O'Leary's emphasis is different from my own. He is interested in the thematics of apocalypticism (constructions of time and evil), whereas I am more concerned with its cultural work (composing individual and communal identities). Nonetheless, his analysis illuminates how the cultural work produces its effects. In the two "frames of acceptance," the tragic plot, thematically constructed around sin and guilt, isolates the evildoer as a victim, while the comic plot, concerned with error, misunderstanding, and ignorance, exposes the evildoer's fallibility and incorporates the evildoer into the community. While such a strict binarism is reductive, it does suggest an interpretive register for performative practices, especially those of queer theater art.[3] Such performative practices constitute the social rituals that compose social identity, the naturalized spectacle in which we are all players. Apocalypticism is conspicuously spectacular, and its first act is often exile.

RITUAL/SPACES

No account of performance is credible unless it takes into account the materiality of space as well as time. In particular, I have in mind Jody Berland's observation that critical theory possesses a "bias toward the temporal" and has "tended to privilege historical determinations in the interpretation of society and culture, and to render spatial determinants as both static and secondary." In trying to account for discourse about AIDS in New York City, I am also aware of the National Research Council's characterization of the city:

> New York is actually a large number of collaborating and competing communities with disparate levels of power and resources. Many of these communities have no direct contact with other communities and compete with each other over resources and entitlements in distant arenas, while others directly confront each other on the streets of the city over specific pieces of turf.[4]

Because of my own familiarity with those neighborhoods in which gay men have become a substantial and visible physical presence, much of this chapter and those that follow are informed by those particular spaces, including Greenwich Village (the West Village and to a lesser extent, the East Village) and Chelsea.

For many gay and lesbian people lower Manhattan has been a promised land or sacred place for much of the twentieth century. While at the turn of the century the Bowery had been a center of "fairy life," in the 1910s and 1920s this honor went to Greenwich Village and Harlem, both the settings of extraordinarily vibrant artistic and cultural activity, with an accompanying openness to bohemian ways of life. As George Chauncey argues, this gay life enjoyed a remarkable degree of visibility and public tolerance, which was admittedly short lived. Social dislocations and the opportunity for new social and erotic relationships during World War II made possible the influx of gay and lesbian people into urban centers where they could develop communal identities, which, though still furtive in many respects, were the foundation of later gay activism and complex forms of gay culture. The material conditions attendant upon the Second World War and the postwar economic expansion made migration into urban centers possible for more gays and lesbians, many of whom experienced urban life for the first time during their military service. It is no coincidence that the two largest ports of embarkation during the war, New York and San Francisco, are today the homes of the largest and most visible gay communities in the United States. The Stonewall riots in the West Village in June 1969 were the culmination of decades of gay lives and cultures, which succeeded in making gay people more visible and audible and in making the Village emblematic of gay life.[5]

Greenwich Village is one of several downtown (the area below 14th Street) Manhattan neighborhoods, though it is usually defined by the East Village and the West Village (Fifth Avenue serves as a dividing line). Originally a village north of the earliest port of New York, its narrow preindustrial streets cut obliquely across the wider right-angled avenues and streets coming from Midtown Manhattan. Stereotypically, the East Village is representative of a younger, hipper, more politically and aesthetically radical population, while the West Village and Chelsea gay residents tend to be older, more affluent, and professional. These characterizations, needless to say, do not do justice to the diversity of these neighborhoods, in terms of race and ethnicity, gender, and social or economic class. The West Village in particular still possesses a kind of cachet as a neighborhood of artists, jazz performers, writers, and bohemians, though inflated property values have tended to keep out the less affluent. Businesses and residences on the Village's side streets are often side by side, creating neighborhood gathering places like bistros, cafes, and taverns, while the city's broader avenues are more exclusively commercial venues.

The 1969 Stonewall Riots were a form of performance in which gay people began to carve out spaces for themselves, a process of renegotiating of space that continues today. During Prohibition, gay venues were as (il)legal as other establishments; but with the end of Prohibition, morality crusades in New York (and elsewhere) legislated prohibitions against taverns owned by or serving a clientele of "perverts and degenerates." As a result, gays who wanted to socialize were at the mercy of bar owners (frequently fronts for organized crime) and the police, who although they were bribed not to do so, occasionally were required to make some show of upholding public morality, a situation that continued into the 1970s. Thus on the night of June 1969, police raided a mob-owned bar, the Stonewall Inn; but this time the patrons fought back.

Even as gay visibility heightened, gay "exiles" required a map or guidebook to the "safe" spaces that gays had appropriated in New York or other cities, thus spawning a guidebook publishing industry. Not only handy to the gay traveler or newcomer, they are a rich historical document for later queer generations, since they chronicle bars, restaurants, sex clubs and emporia, businesses, and public "cruising" spaces. John Francis Hunter's 1971 *The Gay Insider* details New York's gay appropriated venues, such as matinee movie theater balconies, subway station restrooms, parks and the like, in addition to bars and the baths. Hunter also offers cautionary accounts that demonstrate that the Stonewall Riots did not end police harassment of gay space, just gave resistance to it more visibility and credibility. Hunter identifies the portion of the West Village west of Seventh Avenue as "The Casbah," a gay paradise/underworld; the West Village proper, the Gay Capital, whose Christopher Street is "Main Street." Many "orgy bars" were situated in the shabby commercial area, ironically also the location of a literal meat market, the shambles for Manhattan's butchers. The Christopher Street docks on the Hudson River, abandoned when Manhattan lost its preeminence as a seaport, became famous as erotic venues as well. These spaces were the sites of many of the rituals of gay New Yorkers and entered into the lore of gay life nationally, rendering them sacred to those who were composing gay identities. As a result, they were also the sites of negotiation and struggle about a range of queer dissident performances and representations, from public displays of affection, to cross-dressing and nudity, to sexual acts, contests not only between "gays" and "straights" but also among gay people themselves. [6]

EXILE AND PERFORMANCE

Citing an AIDS study by C. E. Rosenberg, the National Research Council's report, *The Social Impact of AIDS in the U.S.*, suggests that "Epidemics appear to have much in common [with each other]. They share a common dramaturgical form of progressive acknowledgment, collective agreement on an explanatory framework, and a negotiated public response."[7] Such a figurative conclusion is highly problematic in that it superimposes a particular "explanatory framework," namely Western dramaturgy with its inevitable trajectory from complication to climax to resolution and denouement, and proceeds to naturalize that trope while essentializing a "natural process" for the material conditions of all epidemics. Nonetheless, this sleight of hand demonstrates the appeal of the dramatic trope and alludes to the performative and spectacular dimensions of such terms

as "plague." Analogously identifying the central characteristic of performance as "restored behavior," Richard Schechner suggests that performance likewise possesses a future (one might say, "apocalyptic") orientation:

> Although restored behavior seems to be founded on past events . . . it
> is in fact [a] synchronic bundle. . . . The past . . . is recreated in terms
> not simply of a present . . . but of a future. . . . This future is the per-
> formance being rehearsed, the "finished thing" to be made graceful
> through editing, repetition, and invention. Restored behavior is both
> teleological and eschatological. It joins first causes to what happens at
> the end of time. It is a model of destiny.[8]

My convergence of the exile trope and apocalyptic performativity
brings onto this stage three cultural productions of the early 1990s that
emerged from gay New Yorkers' catastrophic losses to AIDS during the
preceding decade: Tim Miller's 1992 performance piece, *My Queer Body*;
David Drake's 1992 play *The Night Larry Kramer Kissed Me*; and James
McCourt's 1993 novel, *Time Remaining*. These three texts shared significant
similarities and dissimilarities. Each text featured a solo performer, an
avant-garde cultural role that became more visible during the late 1980s
and early 1990s when some of its practitioners by their frank or startling
representations of the body became embroiled in the conflict over public
funding for the arts. Each also attempted to construct queer origins, a
time *in illo tempore* of both the speaking subject and the gay and lesbian
community; each presented the motif of an exilic landscape and journey
during which the narrator undergoes ordeals (AIDS and homophobia);
and each proposed the grounds for hope in an imaginary queer future.
In addition, Miller's performance piece, Drake's play, and McCourt's
novel explicitly (though not exclusively) addressed a gay male audience
affected by AIDS in order to comfort them and mobilize their action.
However, the two pieces by performance artists and the novel about a
performance artist, were also significantly dissimilar in that their genres—
agitprop performance and stylistically complex novel—encoded both the
material conditions of their production and the intended audiences for
their reception.[9]

Each of these texts interrogated naturalized categories or taxonomies,
through questioning the binarisms that typically establish apocalyptic
discourse, beginning with the literary taxonomies of genre. Miller's and
Drake's performances and McCourt's novel simultaneously were embed-

ded in and resisted the dominant white, Anglo-Saxon, Protestant (or Catholic, in McCourt's case) discourses of their upbringing, a cultural formation that would not be the case, for example, in the similarly apocalyptic *Quotations from a Ruined City*, a piece for several performers by Iranian-born Reza Abdoh and Salar Abdoh.[10] As such, each text explored and privileged notions of identity as performativity in opposition to Western metaphysical conventions of identity as stable essence. The union of Performance Theory and Queer Theory has produced an antiessentialist ontology that examines how concepts of gender and desire have been constructed in Western discourse in an attempt to deconstruct their pernicious effects, particularly upon the bodies of women and sexual dissidents. In "Imitation and Gender Insubordination," Judith Butler asserts that gender is a performance, an imitation without an original; in other words, gender is a "drag." Butler interrogates identity categories in her book *Gender Trouble: Feminism and the Subversion of Identity* in which she asserts that not only gender but biological sex are "regulatory fictions" of oppressive social structures. Butler's work is central to Queer Theory's critique of a Gay/Lesbian Studies methodology that simply reproduces binary oppositions of male/female, masculine/feminine, heterosexual/homosexual. In "Queer Performativity: Henry James's *The Art of the Novel*," Eve Kosofsky Sedgwick responded to Butler and suggested the use of the term "queer performativity" to describe "a strategy for the production of meaning and being in relation to the affect of shame and to the later and related fact of stigma," which she characterized as "simply the first, and remains a permanent, structuring fact of identity."[11]

In a response to Sedgwick, Butler has nuanced her own formulation of performativity "not as self-expression or self-presentation, but as the unanticipated resignifiability of highly invested terms." She has in mind the New York drag "houses" represented in Jenny Livingstone's documentary, *Paris is Burning*. Black and Latino gay men form groups of affiliation that reconfigure, not simply mimic or "do the drag" of "real" families. However, Butler's positive reading of drag performance is at odds with other feminist critics, like Peggy Phelan who critiques drag as a fetishizing of woman, imagining woman without the presence of women: "Gay male cross-dressers *resist* the body of woman even while they make its constructedness visible. This is in part why the misogyny which underlies gay male cross-dressing is so painful to women." Nonetheless, in a discussion of John Epperson's drag persona, "Lypsinka," David Román suggests the tactical usefulness of some drag performance: "Gay men . . . have a long tradition of staging camp as a means to entertain those on the front lines of war." The drag of female impersonation is a contested salient in the discussion of gender and performativity, though not the sole drag, for as RuPaul, "Supermodel of the World," has said, "You're born naked and everything you put on after that is drag."[12]

At the conclusion of his analysis of queer identity and performativity, indebted to Judith Butler's subversive reconstruction of biological sex, Ed Cohen poses a question that, he urges, might pretend a strategic difference in theorizing about sexuality: "How can we affirm a relational and transformational politics of self that takes as its process and its goal the interruption of those practices of differentiation that (re)produce historically specific patterns of privilege and oppression?"[13] Two terms of that query, "interruption" and "transformational," evoke the rhetorical strategy that fantasizes the rupture of history, that imagines ultimate discontinuity or difference, namely apocalyptic discourse, with its millenarian promise of disruption and reversal, which even in its most ideologically pure forms paradoxically predicates that interruption simultaneously upon an external agency outside of human activity (e.g., Judaeo-Christianity's God or Marx's history) and an intentional performance of human agents (e.g., the saved, the workers). Thus, for example, Christian fundamentalists in the 1970s and 1980s contended simultaneously that a future rupture in history was entirely in God's control and that it would be hastened by the toleration of sodomitical performances.

If there are no stable (sexual) identities, no determined "texts" of signifying desires, then apocalyptic discourse might be similarly understood as a performance of desires seeking simultaneously stability and instability, identity and abjection. Thus in the formulation of Pierre Bourdieu the ". . . polysemy of religious language, and the ideological effect of the *unification of opposites* or denial of divisions which it produces, derive from the fact that, at the cost of the *re-interpretations* implied in the production and reception of common language by speakers occupying different positions in the social space, and therefore endowed with different intentions and interests, it manages to speak to all groups and all groups speak it,"[14] thus accounting for apocalyptic tropes among the AIDS-related discourse of both Christian fundamentalists and queer AIDS activists.

David Román asserts that "direct action can result from performance," suggesting the anxiety of many culture workers affected by AIDS who often wonder if "art" contributes to the struggle against

AIDS and homophobia. And Román makes even larger claims for material performances:

> It is by performing all our lives that we produce a chaotic multiplicity of representations, representations that displace, by the very process of proliferation, the authority of a conservative ideology of sexual hegemony, AIDS myths, and aesthetic practices. These endless multiplications and proliferations of difference and confrontation engendered through performance deconstruct oppressive systems of representation and demonstrate the radical capacity of political art in a reactionary, conservative age to both articulate resistance and generate necessary social change.

Román's utopianism finds an ally in Jill Dolan, who asserts:

> Because gay male or lesbian sex is completely out of place—unimaged, unimagined, invisible—in traditional aesthetic contexts, the most transgressive act at this historical moment would be representing it to excess, in dominant and marginalized reception communities. The explicitness of pornography seems the most constructive choice for practicing cultural disruptions.

Isn't it pretty to think so? As a grassroots activist in Virginia, I am aware how paltry the social dividends of queer spectacle, from "RuPaul" to "Ellen," from "Will and Grace" to "Queer As Folk." As a college English professor, I am also conscious how frequently grand are academics' claims for our cultural products. Robert Wallace has wisely observed, "For lesbians and gay men, the production of real intervention—and by this I mean intervention that produces social change—requires the agency of living bodies. Our bodies *are* the issue. How we use them to define and defy the regimes of cultural practice determines the reconstructive moments of our future." Because, as Marvin Carlson observes, the "possibility, even the necessity, of critique if not subversion from within performative activity has become widely accepted, [although] the most effective performance strategies for such subversion remain much debated . . . the subversive possibilities of live performance in itself" are less apparent. My own resistance to the facile equation of visibility with cultural power resonates with Peggy Phelan's cautionary remarks:

> If representational visibility equals power, then almost-naked young white women should be running Western culture. . . . Visibility politics

are additive rather than transformational (to say nothing of revolutionary). They lead to the stultifying "me-ism" to which realist representation is always vulnerable. . . . Visibility politics are compatible with
capitalism's relentless appetite for new markets and with the most satisfying ideologies of the United States: you are welcome as long as you
are productive.

ACT-UP's iconic "Silence = Death" was supplemented with "Action =
Life," but as an academic and an activist I struggle with the next (implied)
supplement, "Discourse (or Performance) = Action" because the product of
cultural work is not always materially evident or incontrovertible. As Phelan
suggests, performance is characterized by its temporality or evanescence.
My attempt here will be to offer a more durable reading of that evanescent
work in, for example, the process of conversion usually signified by "coming out" as it is represented in Miller's, Drake's, and McCourt's texts.[15]

In the last section of this chapter through an historicist/semiotic
critique I want to examine, not what Miller's, Drake's, and McCourt's
performances "might" do—the phantasmic subject of much theoretical
criticism—but what material performances *have actually done* to "inter-
rupt" and "transform" the historically (re)produced patterns of gender/
sexual privilege and oppression (in Cohen's formulation); in other words,
to begin to construct a queer *praxis*. A social semiotic analysis can account for the work produced by each of these three performances, particularly the (re)production of meanings that resist stigmatizing
representations of AIDS and that offer hope for a post-AIDS future.

TIM MILLER'S *MY QUEER BODY*

Tim Miller has been variously compared to an evangelist, a preacher, and
a pastor. Writing for the *Village Voice*, Burt Supree characterized Miller's
audience as "his congregation; he might as well hug and shake hands" and
Miller as "an able preacher, . . . [who] knows just how . . . high he wants to
take us." The reviewer for the *Boston Phoenix* compared Miller's *My Queer
Body* to Dante and Ezekiel and suggested that "if the movement is looking
for an evangelist, here is Miller insisting on celebrating sex." Reviewing
Miller's *Naked Breath* for a California gay and lesbian weekly newspaper,
Kevin Thaddeus Paulson characterized the performer as "[A] queer evan-
gelist. He preaches the gospel of blood and breath and sex that binds us

together. Sex is good." Similarly, the reviewer for the San Diego *Union-Tribune* characterized *Naked Breath* as "a quasi-religious sermonette exhorting gay men to keep up the fierce fight for their rights—and their erotic joy." [16] These critics were not responding to Miller's parody of religious discourse so much as to the fact that Miller, preachers, and evangelical witnesses all present themselves as representative of and for their audiences. Later in this chapter, I will show how Miller shares this method of representation with David Drake and with James McCourt's characters. Like North America's colonial and early republican Methodist circuit riders, Miller is an itinerant "preacher." Though "home" is currently Santa Monica, California, he maintains a wide-ranging performance schedule.

Miller articulated a spirituality for his work in the essay "Jesus and the Queer Performance Artist," included in a collection edited by Malcolm Boyd and Nancy L. Wilson, *Amazing Grace: Stories of Lesbian and Gay Faith*. He characterizes his work as referring ". . . in very different ways to Christian imagery and archetypes as a way of exposing and healing the lies and hurt of our society." Ironically, when Miller came under attack from the Christian Right through its point man, Jesse Helms, Miller was exploring performance and liturgy He experienced a self-described "exile from [his] . . . Christian self" while finding again and again that Christian symbols inform his work: "crucifixion and rebirth, conflict and communion, epiphany and despair. The desire for moments of peace. Sorrow about the sadness of the world. A radical desire to ease suffering, my own and others.' " Miller's spirituality is informed by a profound contradiction. Taking into consideration, "the blandness of organized suburban Christianity" (Miller's California Congregationalist roots), the church's history of inquisition and oppression, and his postmodern consciousness, Miller concludes, "Nothing personal, Jesus. I just can't stand the company you keep. It seemed to make more sense to chuck the whole thing." However, the more formative childhood faith pressed him: "The first man I was ever in love with was Jesus. He was sweet. He was strong. He didn't play football or scream at me and he wore great clothes." To some extent he was able to reconcile this contradiction by imagining "Jesus as activist . . . Jesus as a member of ACT UP" and "[t]he crucifixion as the ultimate civil disobedience." In this way Miller attempted to construct a spirituality that was both affective or contemplative/mystical as well as activist.[17]

According to Weinstein, Miller's "voice is pointedly addressed to queers; by anyone else, he is overheard" a point that Miller would agree with in regard to his New York audiences, but not in the other venues where he has performed. Some reviewers, like Kevin Thaddeus Paulson and Robert Nesti, have tendentiously slighted Miller's (and other performance artists') work as "preaching to the choir," a characterization that Miller has challenged eloquently with coauthor David Román in an article arguing in favor of "preaching to the converted . . . first as a descriptive which names the potential affinities between the two terms of its locution—preacher/congregation, performer/audience; second (however much it historically has been deployed as a derogatory), as a descriptive for community-based, and often community-specific, lesbian and gay theatre and performance." Miller explicitly acknowledged the roots of the solo performance tradition in the American oratorical tradition, including Baptist preaching. Therefore, Miller viewed his "preaching" as a form of activism that is "creating a sense of community, helping people to survive" and "entertaining the troops or cheerleading."[18] Although the assertion of a community of the "converted" naively creates a binarism (i.e., the converted/the unconverted) that ignores the instability of any identity and in particular the vulnerability of queer identity in the face of heterocentric domination, the gay or lesbian "converted":

> [N]eeds to be understood as a dynamic assembly that both individually and communally enters into the space of performance to sustain the very state of conversion. Truth be told, however, the converted are never wholly converted. Rather, like the process of coming out, which is a lifelong project of continuous self-identification and revelations, there is no definitive moment of absolute conversion. Instead, to be among the converted is to be open to a series of conversions, it is a way of being that implies a constant state of negotiation and need depending on the specific psychosocial and sociohistorical occasions of our daily lives. Conversion, understood from this perspective, demands a continual testing of one's identity, if only as a means to affirm it.

Miller also decried what he saw as the academics' separation of sacred storytelling from theatre and the "schism of spirit from the theatre," and he affirmed that "Queer theatre, like all theatre, is about conversion and transformation," experiences which require regular "revival" (in both the theatrical and religious senses of that term).[19] Much as Ed Cohen and Judith Butler argue about a subject's gender and sexual identity, the performance audience or "community" (admitting the ambiguous and overdetermined character of that term and the disparateness and temporality of the reality it signifies) rehearses and "plays" or "pretends" rather than "achieves" its identity: coming into close physical contact with other audience members, responding to performers as a group of addressed subjects, identifying with the subjects of the performance, meeting old friends or making new acquaintances, savoring the pleasures of having "made the scene" of a talked-about show or performance, and discussing or remembering the performance during intermission or after the theater.

Community-based performance artists or "solo performers" (the term Miller prefers) "reclaim the once-longstanding alliance between performers and spectators as members of community who, in the enactment of communal ritual, enable the power of individuals to gather and perform the necessary constitutive rehearsal of identity."[20] For New York gay men particularly, in a city where "the theatre" is both a major local industry and an iconic gay workplace, public theatrical spaces become ritual spaces that are attended regularly, one might almost say, "faithfully." In New York, at the same time, homo- and heterosexual eroticism become public spectacles or theater: the hunky Calvin Klein model clad only in briefs hovers over Times Square; male construction workers whistle and call to female office workers on the sidewalk; sex workers perform on stage in theaters; men seek other men in the Rambles of Central Park, at the bathhouse, or on the theatrically lighted dance floors. Even if one is not a direct participant in such activities, the New Yorker is inevitably drawn vicariously into the city's erotic theatricality. As Andrew Holleran has written about sex between men in the darkened Metropolitan cinema, "It's a form of theater . . . the final testimony to this performance the fact that he can leave now, he has got what he came for, and needed. Ah, New York: always the same, ever new."[21]

Tim Miller's overt acknowledgment of sexuality in performance pieces made him the target of attacks from the political and religious right, including Senator Jesse Helms whose criticisms of funding that Miller received from the National Endowment for the Arts prompted then NEA director John Frohnmyer in 1990 to withdraw grants to Miller and three other artists, which provoked a successful lawsuit by the artists.[22] In the middle of *My Queer Body*, for example, Miller stripped before recounting episodes of antigay violence or the depredations of AIDS, sat naked on an audience member's lap, and later addressed his own exposed penis, which he remonstrated for not "performing" on cue. Obviously taken out of context (the tactic of demagogues like Helms and Donald Wildmon), these details of Miller's performances may seem at best sensational. For hip theater-goers, however, stage nudity evokes a tradition on American stage going back at least to the experimental theater of the 1960s or more mainstream productions like *Oh, Calcutta!* and *Hair*, for gay men in New York, a slender attractive youthful male sitting on an audience member's lap summoned up the dancing hustlers in theaters around Times Square (before it was Disneyfied in the 1990s), go-go bars, or frenzied Saturday nights dancing at The Saint. Yet as Jack Anderson pointed out in a review of *My Queer Body*, adverting to Miller's self-described spirituality, this performance is anything but salacious. Rather, Miller confronted his audience with the sheer physicality of the body, site of both pleasure and pain; the site of loss (for example the death of a lover, the end of a relationship), paradoxically, can also become the site of consolation (the embrace of a friend, orgasm). At the same time he was forcing his audiences to acknowledge that the "culture war" in the contemporary United States was not a war of ideas but of control of the body.[23]

My Queer Body took an audience on a journey from Miller's own origins *in illo tempore* through tribulation and testing to a proleptic fantasy of a queer utopia. Miller entered behind the audience, a "rear entry" that he acknowledged as both an erotic and liturgical pun, summoned the bodies of those who had gathered in that space, and began to narrate his own conception, his young parents making love on a bed that would be passed on to him as an adolescent and would be the site of his first lovemaking. Miller described how he met and spent the day with Robert, the boy who would be his first love. An auto accident intervenes in the idyll, but the proximity to danger brings Tim and Robert closer seeking consolation and the two boys spend the night at Tim's, sharing "The best thing we get while we're in our bodies on the planet Earth" (320). Miller read his own body spatially: "My skin is a map. A map of my world. My secret world. It tells you where I've been. And how to get to where I come from. . . . I go on journeys." (321).

At that point in the performance, the piece, now set in the present, took a more explicitly apocalyptic turn: "There is a plague and hatred on the land. An earthquake within. Whole continents have been lost to us. . . . Then the burning began. . . . Burned up my city of angels" (321–22). During a demonstration at the Los Angeles County Museum of Art, Tim is beaten by police, but escapes to a Denny's restaurant, where a waitress becomes an attending angel who sends Tim into the Mojave desert and a vision at the Amboy volcano crater. In this vision he stripped off his clothes (which the performing Miller actually did as he relates the vision), recalled the violence of nuclear anxiety, consumer excess, and homophobia; he watched friends and lovers die. Miller narrated how a horrible beast crawled into the crater, clawing at him and pulling friends and lovers out of Miller's rectum. But at this juncture, Miller announced, "I made that all up. All about the volcano and the beast. I lied to you. I'm sorry. Don't hate me. I don't really know what's in my volcano" (325). Miller typically resisted climax or catharsis, the politics-as-usual of Western drama. Furthermore, he acknowledged that all he knows is his own physical presence, which he makes more real to the audience by walking naked around them, finally sitting in the lap of one audience member into whose eyes he looks to see his own reflection, a significant gesture of identity.[24]

Miller then addressed his own penis, demanding that it "GET HARD!" though the recalcitrant member was unresponsive, requiring Miller to finish his mythmaking: "You say not until I finish my story? OK. This is a fairy tale. Maybe I can make up a new ending and maybe we'll find our way out of the volcano" (328). In this fantasy, Miller returned to the demonstration at the Museum of Art ("Fuck this Jungian mythopoetic stuff. My queer friends are getting beat up back at the museum" [330]), the demonstrators force the governor out of office, and the marginalized make important advances into the new millennium, including electing a black lesbian president, who appoints Miller performance artist laureate. During the performance he invited the audience to help him make the inauguration performance piece. To the accompaniment of Ravel's "Bolero," Miller described the ritual of performing sex as "a special moment. A sacrament of sorts. Made more sacred for our fears. . . . This is the promised land." (333, 334). The erotic exploration of two naked bodies, and metaphorically the exploration of performer and audience, entails an intersubjective construction of identity: "Naked in the sight of each other. The only ones that matter. I am fucking, I am being fucked. Touched and touching. Time now to know each other and ourselves" (335). Like the Christian Book of Revelation, Miller's narrative fantasy ended with a marriage: "But, now, I feel the blessing of being closer than they told us was possible. The fuckers lied to us. I am not ashamed of nakedness and I will not [be] cast out of paradise by right-wing bigots or some fucking hunky archangel with a flaming sword in some garden. This is one sex between two queer men's bodies in the time of trial on the planet Earth at the very end of the second millennium" (336).

Although employing apocalyptic tropes—beasts, catastrophe, defilement, sacred eros—Miller was also repudiating the apocalyptic trajectory, first by discarding a narrative climax's closure, then by rescripting the Western mythos of the Fall—the event upon which apocalyptic closure is predicated—by refusing to leave the Garden in the first place. Miller's parodic apocalypse allowed him to present the audience with recognizable Western figures by which he could ridicule celebrity homophobes and provide imaginative future possibilities. For example, in the opening "cosmogonic" battle narrative, Tim's spunky "queer little spermlet" fights sperm that look like Jesse Helms, the Joint Chiefs of Staff, and gay bashers. The identification of these sperm differed from performance to performance in order to include local or topical references. For Miller the sacred dimensions of sex deploy more than consolation, though certainly nonetheless consoling; sex mobilizes:

> It's like this sex will revive the big identity document that says, 'I am! My body belongs to me!' Flipping the bird to fear. Because even though there has been so much death, we are still here with our skin and bones. There is blood and spirit and queer horndogginess within and about me. Between you and me. Between your butts and your seats. Between our hearts and our heads. (334)

According to Miller, "[T]his kind of art is about creating a sense of community, helping people survive. . . . I want to gather the audience, and bring them with me on a journey of pleasure, love and loss." Miller's work, like that of the typical apocalyptist, arose out of what he called "communities of crisis"; he intended to intervene in the "real war going on around the soul of all kinds of things," though he recognized the strategic limitations of those interventions.[25]

During much of the 1980s, the audience or "community of crisis" for Miller was composed of the many gay men who came to see him and others perform at New York's East Village Performance Space 122, an alternative performance venue that Miller cofounded with Charles Moulton and Charles Dennis. At the performance Beth Goodman attended, she was "one of the only women in the audience; most of the others were box office employees and stage crew. The audience was composed almost exclusively of men, mostly gay and some, presumably (an unfortunate safe guess in the East Village), HIV positive."[26] Miller has noted that audience responses to his work were conditioned by both the character of local queer communities, the availability of alternative performance traditions, and the type of space in which he performed.[27] The informality of P.S. 122, the audience of East Village and "theater types" who frequently attended its performances, and the availability of a wide range of performance forms and spaces (basement clubs, warehouses, small theaters, and the like) for gay men in New York, produce a savvy audience, for whom this converted grade school may also have been the site of workshops and sex parties, in addition to performances, thus in Miller's assessment a "highly consecrated" space where "people had transformative experiences."[28] His visibility as a local activist lent credibility to his function as a solo performer; and the work done at P.S. 122 was widely publicized. Insofar as he is also a gay performer deliberately playing to an audience of gay men, Miller's sexy queer body can also be read semiotically: lean, boyish, smooth-chested, and well-endowed, with dark curly hair, dressed in the Queer Nation uniform of the late 1980s and early 90s (black Doc Martin boots or black Converse high-tops, ripped jeans, tank top shirt, plumbing chains around the neck), Miller is the swarthy troublemaker your mother liked but nonetheless didn't want you to become. He is the boy who initiated you into sex.

DAVID DRAKE'S *THE NIGHT LARRY KRAMER KISSED ME*

In contrast to Miller's punk darkness, David Drake's body signifies ephebic ingenuousness, characterized by Sylvie Drake in her review of the play as "boyishness and biceps" with "darting eyes . . . litheness."[29] Drake is an self-acknowledged sissy, the golden boy of the neighborhood, the blue-eyed, blond "best little boy in the world" who journeyed from his Baltimore home to New York in order to be a bad little boy. His 1992 one-actor play, *The Night Larry Kramer Kissed Me* concerned this journey and projected Drake's "Everyman" character (whom stage directions in the published text characterize generically as the "Performer") into a postmillennial future, after a gay revolution and a cure for AIDS.

The play began in a section subtitled "The Birthday Triptych" with Drake's queer *in illo tempore*, his sixth birthday, June 27, 1969, the night of the Stonewall riots and coincidentally the first time he went to the theater, attending the Baltimore Community Theater's production of Leonard Bernstein's *West Side Story*. The play then moved exactly ten years later to Drake's first date with another boy whom he takes to see the musical *Pippin* (a scene that leads inadvertently to his parents' discovery that he is gay), and eventually leads to his twenty-second birthday in 1985, when he attended a performance of Larry Kramer's *The Normal Heart*, Drake's eponymous "kiss."

The play then advanced along a series of vignettes or episodes, that concerned working out at the gym, personals ads, AIDS activism, and a vision of a utopian future. Paralleling the journey from "best little (sissy) boy in the world" to out queer sissy boy is Drake's movement from AIDS-related grief to rage, from fear to courage. Initially running "to escape the invisible, unprintable killer stalking" him (17) through the escapism of Broadway musicals, Drake eventually came to recognize in gay men's gym workout routines not only an erotic purpose but also a militant one as well:

> We're-to-build-our-selves-for-hands-on-war
> our-bo-dies-are-our-weap-ons-for
> the-day-we-bash-the-bash-ers-back
> in-to-the-graves-they've-dug-for-us
> so-we-can-have-the-fin-al-laugh
> when-we-sit-back-&-tell-the-lore
> of-how-we-won-the-final-war . . .
> pressing-towards-the-day-we-win-the
> FI-
> NAL-
> WAR-
> FROM-
> GO-
> ING-
> TO-
> THE GYM. (42)

These lines were delivered in the rhythm of a military jogging drill that eventually turned into a four-beat march cadence.

Following an elegiac account of friends and a lover who had died and a repudiation of musicals' escapism, a section that ended in Drake's character's entry into AIDS activism, the play concluded with a proleptic fantasy set in 1999 on New Year's Eve. The performer and his mate are spending the evening alone, having watched a queer remake of the Robert Redford/Barbara Streisand film, *The Way We Were*. In addition to the new year, they are celebrating the first anniversary of their Legal Domestic Partnership, remembering the doting attention of both sets of parents at the "Celebration Party at the Queer Pier Dance Hall on Lake Erie. Buffalo—that's where Bill's family lives" (80). Their "wedding" completes a period of militant gay activism, including a '96 Pentagon Action and a Together We'll Take Manhattan Action, the Queer War of '96 which ends with AIDS-researcher Robert Gallo (who falsely claimed to have discovered HIV), antifeminist Phyllis Schlafly, and conservative congressman William Dannemeyer in prison, former New York mayor Ed Koch and NIH administrator Anthony Fauci exiled in South America, and Rush Limbaugh assassinated. The performer prophesied a Queer Cultures Wing added to the Smithsonian, the inclusion of "sexual orientation" on the federal census survey forms, and the outing of Siskel and Ebert. More bleakly, he also admonished Chicago, San Francisco, L.A., Dallas, Atlanta, D.C., Boston (the names of the cities could be tailored to the theater venue): "[G]et prepared . . . 'cause the blood and fire will tear through your cities" (84).

According to Drake's introduction, the play represented his own movement toward the formation of an individual queer identity that eventually led him "to bonding with my tribe" (xiv). The personal is the communal insofar as coming out, acknowledging the goodness of queer sexuality, is a "quest" that grounds the "hope to find [an] emotional and spiritual kinship to other gay and lesbian people" (xii). In an "Author's Note" Drake constructed a version of that group identity that paralleled his own coming of age and initiation into queer identity; this communal identity, like the individual's, was understood as narrative: "In hearing their stories, we begin to understand the experience, strength, and hope that have distinguished a people's shape, depth, and direction. These stories, if told truthfully, also hold answers and knowledge that can serve as guideposts for the future" (89). Drake was therefore concerned to construct a myth of origins: Stonewall as the birth of "modern" gay activism; a production of *West Side Story* by queer composer Bernstein as the consecratory moment of Drake's queerness, paradigmatically represented as a conversion or "born-again" experience; the characterization of David Summers as "the first person ever arrested in the name of AIDS activism" (90), and so forth.[30] This myth of origins was even reproduced in the play's production history, opening in 1992 a few days before Drake's birthday and the Stonewall anniversary, and closing on the night of those anniversaries in 1993. Nonetheless, attempting to resist the essentialist tendencies of such myths, Drake underscored in his introduction to the play the performativity of gay identity: "Getting out of the closet is a journey in and of itself. Staying out is another. But where do you go from there? Where is 'out'? What are the obstacles that you face? Where do they come from? How do you overcome them? What is the

source of your commitment to staying out? How deep does it run?" (xii).
Like Tim Miller and David Román, Drake acknowledged this identity as
a continuing process. And his "finale" was not final; resisting closure,
Drake represented the unfinished business of queer activism, even in a
utopian future that recognizes gay marriage.

The apocalyptic trajectory from exile to marriage, the comic outcome of the Book of Revelation in the wedding of the Bride and the
Lamb (Rev. 21), also marked Drake's bourgeois position and constructed
an audience bent on affectional assimilation rather than erotic dissent. If
eroticism led Drake into activism—he attended his first ACT-UP meeting after picking up an activist—it does not do so with the same Dionysian
tonalities of Miller's *My Queer Body*. In the final vignette Drake domesticated the erotic charge built up in the earlier "12" Single" scene by
fantasizing a society tolerant of domesticated homo-affectionalism:

> And you'll see people like Bill and me—out, together, walking hand
> in hand down the streets of New York . . . Toledo . . . Portland, Rich-
> mond, Raleigh, Tallahassee, Albuquerque, New Mexico; Morgantown,
> West Virginia; Pomona [again, the names can be tailored to the the-
> ater venue] . . . without condemnation, restrictions, compromises, or
> closets. (85)

These couples, however, were not sexual outlaws or erotic prophets.

Drake's concern for the performance's accessibility to a "mainstream"
audience was evident in the Anchor Books edition of the play where
Drake offered a gloss on its topical references, suggesting a desire to make
the play intelligible to non-New York gay men or to nongay New Yorkers. The play's director, Chuck Brown, confirmed this intention when he
characterized the play's varied audiences: "We have gotten letters from
people all over the country who have been in New York to see the
play. . . . They are thrilled, frightened and empowered by seeing gay life
on stage." These audiences also included "more enlightened" theater goers
and those seeking a production with "underground" cachet and " 'cute
straight couples from Westchester.' "[31]

Unlike Miller's performance, Drake's in *The Night Larry Kramer Kissed
Me* was reviewed in the mainstream *Time* magazine.[32] Further, his vita in
the published edition of the play noted his prior roles in *Pageant* (as Miss
Deep South) and Charles Busch's drag comedy *Vampire Lesbians of Sodom*,
as well as television and film appearances, all of which taken together

constructed a professional identity that was both impeccable and off-beat without being controversial. Drake was not on a Helms or NEA hit list. Both Drake's professional persona and the stage persona shied away from erotic radicalism, preferring instead to appropriate bourgeois heterosexual relations, including references to the kitsch *The Way We Were* and the sentimental "Auld Lang Syne," gay marriage and weddings, and a people's rebellion in the solidarity of gay and AIDS organizations with NOW, NAACP, ACLU, and AFL-CIO. This fantastic solidarity imagined breaking through gay/straight binary categories in a nonerotic marriage of populist politics that contrasted with the third section's ("Why I Go to the Gym") binarisms of boy/man, Us/Them, and gay/straight.

And in a sense, the seventh and last section fulfills the prophecy of the third section, ". . . so-we-can-have-the-fin-al-laugh/when-we-sit-back-&-tell-the-lore/of-how-we-won-the-final-war," in its comedic, last-laugh nuptial resolution. This representation of an end-time without a stable resolution moved scholar-critic Richard Dellamora to write:

> When I saw the play, the final section galvanized the audience, for a moment, into a community. It was a curious sensation: to hear unfolded before one a fiction of the future that expressed unformulated wishes as though they were accomplished facts, at once private, secure, and shared. . . . Mortal closure gives way to (a proleptic recollection of) possibility. The structure also does political work, reminding listeners, queer, straight, or otherwise, that "the first resurrection" is still around the corner.[33]

What is remarkable to me about Dellamora's impression is that it evokes indirectly the play's simultaneous desire for closure ("accomplished facts . . . secure, and shared") and its resistance to closure ("still around the corner"), its antiapocalyptic millennialism. That is, Drake employed figures of apocalyptic hope and bliss while refusing those of apocalyptic disaster.

Drake argued an apocalypse, with its trajectory of future fulfillment and promise of a conjugal or erotic last laugh, not to assert an essential, determined future, but to galvanize (in Dellamora's terms) a provisional community in the present, a performative identity whose existence was precisely its performative elusiveness, so aptly described in Peggy Phelan's feminist formulation:

> Performance's only life is in the present. Performance cannot be saved, recorded, documented, or otherwise participate in the circulation of

representations *of* representations: once it does so, it becomes something other than performance. To the degree that performance attempts
to enter the economy of reproduction it betrays and lessens the promise
of its own ontology. Performance's being, like the ontology of subjectivity proposed here, becomes itself through disappearance.

As Phelan notes, performance criticism is thus paradoxically thrown into
question, since it can only be a symptom of the desire for something that
is not real. She redeems critical work, however, by asserting that "feminist
critical writing is an enactment of belief in a better future; the act of
writing brings that future closer." Identifying two anchor points for performance in a body Real and a psychic Real, Phelan can write of "the
hope we fake and perform and the hope we thereby make and have.
Hope's power is measured in this faking. Each performance registers how
much we want to believe what we know we see is not all we really have,
all we really are."[34] The substance of things unseen. Both Tim Miller's *My
Queer Body* and David Drake's *The Night Larry Kramer Kissed Me* attempted to construct provisional or tactical identities (the performer's,
the audience's) in the present to extrapolate future strategic possibilities.

However, formal similarities between Miller's and Drake's performances mask an economic or material difference in their production,
which Alisa Solomon noted "has everything to do with the form and
politics of the shows." Although Tim Miller told me that he found
invidious the negative comparisons between his work and Drake's, he
acknowledged that his own work requires his physical presence (and thus
he generally does not give permission for another performer to present
his material),[35] whereas Drake's was deliberately positioned by producer
Sean Strub (a successful gay-community marketing entrepreneur) as a
play, rather than a performance piece, in order to attract newspaper
reviews and a more mainstream audience. The venues of each differed as
well. Drake performed *The Night Larry Kramer Kissed Me* in the West
Village's Perry Street Theatre, a remodeled space equipped with standard
theatre hardware; Miller, in the appropriated and intimate space of the
East Village's P.S. 122. With its fairly complex design and lighting and
sound cues, Drake's required more theatrical resources than Miller's agitprop performances. Drake's also required an extended run in order to
recoup its costs, whereas Miller could perform his once or twice in one
location before moving on. Drake's play's budget of $110,000 (recouped
in less than six months), of which $45,000 was spent on marketing,

would pay for fifteen productions for three years at the WOW Cafe or over 200 of Miller's productions. However, as Alisa Solomon noted, developing a crossover play requires more than marketing and a budget; the performance must also accommodate a mixed audience, and her criticism is that Drake's vision of queer Armageddon did not "envision any profound reordering. Drake's radicalism remains thin, naive, unthreatening." Like radioactive dye, Solomon's critique reveals a fracture within New York's communities of sexual dissent, the growing rupture through the 1980s of another binary opposition, this one between "gay" and "queer," the first predicated on the homo/hetero binarism; the second, on its deconstruction. In Solomon's reading, Miller's queer politics resisted the assimilation into middle-class culture that Drake's seemed to woo.

In an article for *Theater* Peggy Phelan had a different take on Miller. First, Phelan proposed that the "dramatic tension of *My Queer Body* is located in Miller's three minutes invocation to his penis." If I did not know Peggy Phelan, I would be tempted to guess that she was a gay man obsessed with dick. However, her comment on the semiotics of Miller's body—"But for me, somehow, good looks, boyish charm, and perfect intentions are not, in and of themselves, the stuff of progressive representation"—would have scotched that notion. I have seen *My Queer Body* and studied its written text but cannot see Miller's addressing his penis as the center of the performance's "dramatic tension," which instead seems to occur just prior when he sits naked in an audience member's lap:

> This is the most nervous part of the performance. Here, feel my heart. I see my face reflected in your eyes. I am here with you. I *am* here with you. My body is right here. You are right there. Here, feel my heart. I still feel alone. A little afraid of all of you. And I could tell you another sweet or a scary story like I've tried to do tonight. But whatever I did . . . it would be a lot wetter and messier and human and complicated than when I stand up there naked in the red theatrical light and pretend I'm going into the volcano. (Miller 326)

Miller's peroration to his penis that followed serves two purposes: it ironically undercut the potential erotic sentimentality of his nakedness and it served as a trope for erotic activism. Second, Phelan was disappointed that Miller did not explore "a newer, broader notion of sociality and identity," but for many queer men the social barriers militating against male-male intimacy are continuously reproduced and policed in our daily lives, and thus Miller's performance modeled an alternative sociality. He was, after all, performing "*My*" *Queer Body*, not "*Our*" *Queer Bodies*. Finally, Phelan was dismayed that Miller's "most radical 'alternative' vision of political utopia is that of himself performing at the inaugural celebration of the president of the United States . . . a black lesbian. . . . The notion of a queer body here . . . is predicated on maintaining powerful lesbians (of all colors) as the stuff of fantasy—comic or paranoid. And that's not queer—that's business as usual."[36]

The reception of Miller's and Drake's performances was varied and complex, caught up in audiences' insatiable, competing desires for stability and for tricking stability, and not simply because of differing ideologies. Similarly, the differing material conditions of performances (like location and audience demographics) affected the ways in which the performers' words and bodies were "read," as Carlson suggests:

> The movement of lesbian and gay performance away from audiences identified with those subcultures into more heterogeneous reception situations has opened much more complex questions of how to negotiate appropriation, display, and representation that is politically and socially responsible. The activity of the performer is no longer the central concern of speculation on this phenomenon. It is rather the interplay of performer and public.

Like our national apocalyptic rituals, their performances tended to construct an end, and then to deconstruct it, out of the discursive materials already at hand. Richard Schechner contends that:

> Restored behavior is symbolic and reflexive: not empty but loaded behavior multivocally broadcasting significances. These difficult terms express a single principle: The self can act in/as another; the social or transindividual self is a role or a set of roles. Symbolic and reflexive behavior is the hardening into theater of social, religious, aesthetic, medical, and educational process. Performance means: never for the first time. It means: for the second to the nth time. Performance is "twice-behaved behavior."

Resisting the seductions of apocalypticism, performance also means "never for the last time." If that is the case for the ephemeral live performance, it is more so with writing and the printed text in which readerly performance can resist the sense of an ending.[37]

WRITING IS A DRAG: JAMES MCCOURT'S *TIME REMAINING*

In the first two instances, I have written about performers whose language, at second hand, is recorded on a typeset page (in addition to the counterfeit of the performances on videotapes). The scripts of *My Queer Body* or *The Night Larry Kramer Kissed Me* and the videotapes of specific performances are phantoms, much like the other signifiers we use in the West to indicate the subject. The intersubjectivity of performance is utterly absent as is the physical space of its occurrence. Whereas I am a participant in the live performance, I am a voyeur in its print or media reproduction.

Now, however, I write about a performance that only exists as writing on the typeset page, James McCourt's third novel, *Time Remaining*. In this case I recall Peggy Phelan's observation that "[t]he challenge raised by the ontological claims of performance for writing is to re-mark again the performative possibilities of writing itself. The act of writing toward disappearance, rather than the act of writing toward preservation, must remember that the after-effect of disappearance is the experience of subjectivity itself." At the same time as she attributes the performativity of writing, she reminds us that "Writing, an activity which relies on the reproduction of the Same . . . for the reproduction of meaning, can broach the frame of performance but cannot mimic an art that is nonreproductive." So while the reception regimes of the written text and of the performance already differ, indeed in some ways oppose each other, I want to look at them as Robert Hodge suggests, "as different orientations to a common object, consisting of meanings that both link and oppose verbal text (script) and performance text (theatrical action)."[38]

Time Remaining is likely to be categorized as a novel, composed as it is of a shorter and a longer prose fiction or tale. However, several critics have registered its theatricality. Pearl Bell noted "its extravagant, playful, anti-serious theatricality . . . its reliance on travesty, impersonation, artifice" and less enthusiastically as "McCourt's intermittently brilliant, often boring performance of the 'melodrama of remembering.' " Wayne Koestenbaum has characterized the McCourt of his first novel as the "novelist as diva," a trope that Bertha Harris extended in her review of *Time Remaining*: "Mr. McCourt's 'oltrano' voice (the unsurpassed range of Mawrdew, diva of divas) continues to ravish us with our old favorites. . . . And the drag his intrepid characters wear in this first of Mr. McCourt's explicitly gay fictions is as resplendent as the writing" adding that McCourt's characterizations produce "bravura arias." The performativity of the characters mirrors and feeds back the performativity of the writer's writing of the characters; both the characters and the writer are in drag: the first sartorial, the second verbal.[39]

In the first section of *Time Remaining*, "I Go Back to the Mais Oui," Danny Delancey—performance artist, female impersonator, and veteran of the outrageous Eleven Against Heaven—offers a monologue on New York gay life from the 1950s. One night after a performance of this monologue, Delancey is joined on the last train to his Long Island home by Danny "Odette" O'Doyle, transvestite ballerina, autodidact polymath, and recent executor of the ashen remains of eight members of the Eleven Against Heaven, depositing them in the various sacred rivers and other waters of Europe; the second, longer portion of the book—"A Chance to Talk"—recounts their conversation on the milk train. The Eleven Against Heaven were a band of drag queens whose earlier incarnation had been in McCourt's first novel, *Mawrdew Czgowchwz* (1975), where they were the "Secret Seven" fans of the eponymous "oltrano" diva. Many of this first novel's characters returned a decade later in McCourt's second book-length fiction, *Kaye Wayfaring in "Avenged"* (1984), as some of *Time Remaining*'s do in his later, *Delancey's Way* (2000).[40]

These four books are tied together by more than reappearing characters since time is a preoccupation of each. *Mawrdew Czgowchwz* begins: "There was a time (time out of mind) in the eternal progress of *divadienst*, at that suspensory pause in its career just prior to the advent of what was to be known as 'Mawrdolatry' "; the second, *Kaye Wayfaring in "Avenged"*: "Sitting shivering in time, Kaye Wayfaring brooded"; the fourth, *Delancey's Way*: "I never went to bed early in my life. Until a minute ago . . ." In addition to its title, *Time Remaining* announces its preoccupation with time in its introductory epigraph from poet James Schuyler: "A few days are all we have. So count them as they pass." At its conclusion the novel also resists apocalyptic ruptures in time: "And that's why I suppose I feel my story won't end crashed into a wall. Is that an Allegory?" Perhaps not, but McCourt is attuned to narrative structures of myth and romance.

McCourt has said that in *Time Remaining* he is "adapting the medieval troubadour quest stories, like Sir Gawain and the Green Knight and the legend of Parsifal, to our [gay] tradition. You see, Odette is on a quest, too." Numerous critics have characterized the book as Joycean, and McCourt finds this comparison apt: "Both [*Ulysses* and *Time Remaining*] . . . are about journeys, and both end with sleep." McCourt's streams of monologue are likewise reminiscent of the Dubliner's. Odette, the

voracious reader, is alert to the Homeric Ulysses when she tells Delancey,
"I remember that after I finished every Oz book there was, I picked up
the *Odyssey*—purely because of the homonym: I figured if it *sounded* like
Oz, it might—and, of course, it did," a bit of un-Bloomian (Harold, not
Leopold) canon-busting in which Miss Dorothy Gale of Kansas meets
Odysseus of Ithaca in the pantheon of heroic literature.[41]

   Time Remaining is Joycean in more than its stream of consciousness
form and its verbal and narrative playfulness; McCourt's allusive style is
at its most virtuosic in this third book, which tends to exclude from its
reading community those who are not adepts in opera, cinematic trivia,
Irish Catholicism, and the New York cabaret circuit. Even some members
of the gay men's book group that I belong to, for example, found the
book frequently obscure and inaccessible, despite our numbers' including
college professors, a psychiatrist, an ex-priest, and a hair stylist, "types"
you would ordinarily assume to be among the queer cognoscenti. By
excluding some readers, these allusions construct a reading community
with shared values, interests, and history, specifically (mostly white and
middle-class) urban gay men at midlife who have (so far) survived despite
having done it all and seen it all. However, exclusion alone does not
construct a community; others are included by their ability to "read":

> So the "in-jokes," the "secret" codes, the iconography of dress, move-
> ment, and speech which can be read by those within the community,
> but escape the interpretive power of those external to it, can create
> another expressive language which cannot be translated by those who
> are not familiar with the meanings of this intimate tongue.[42]

In part, these codes may mark an older generation of gay men, in midlife or beyond, for whom negotiating public space and reconfiguring it
into safer gay space required less ostensible signification. There is also the
sheer pleasure of auditioning a performance of verbal wit and camp
allusion, even when we do not "get" all the references.[43]

   Gay camp may codify an older generation's configuration of deviant
sexuality. In " 'It's My Party and I'll Die If I Want To!': Gay Men, AIDS,
and the Circulation of Camp in U.S. Theater," David Román offers this
reading of performer John Epperson's character, "Lypsinka":

> For many gays, especially those who are older, Epperson brings up a
> familiar and important style, which may have lost its initial potency and
> immediate urgency. While the gay bar along with drag entertainment has

long been essential for gays (and lesbians) as a refuge from the culture of the closet, since Stonewall gay men have had many more options for meeting and communicating. Furthermore, the social spaces where drag and camp were first assigned have expanded so that camp culture has now permeated the mainstream. Thus, Lypsinka (re)occupies that place in gay culture, and (re)provides that once flourishing space for gay men. [Epperson's] *I Could Go On Lip-Synching* serves as a fantasy for a certain gay spectatorship yearning for the "simplicity" of life before AIDS. . . . In many ways, Lypsinka's coded and specialized iconography and vocabulary validate the subject position of mainly older white gay male spectators.[44]

This nostalgia is not only for a less dangerous biomedical "past" before AIDS but also for an idealized binary gender-role regime in which men's knowledge consisted in strength, women's in elegance. This fantasy also has appeal for those of us who fuel that eternal consumption engine called the Baby Boomers, for whom a mystique of the 1950s and 1960s, the historical period before our fall into the complexities of sexuality, is still quite powerful.

I saw this glamour at work in June 1994 during the twenty-fifth anniversary Stonewall celebration in New York City when I was in the audience for Charles Busch's *Dressing Up! The Ultimate Dragfest*, a one-night performance that featured such stellar drags as Charles Pierce, Milton Berle and, of course, Busch himself, among others. In addition to the Imperial Court of New York, the large mainstream cross-dressing "house," the audience was filled with drags young and old. But what was striking was the number of men in our thirties, forties, and fifties for whom television's "Uncle Miltie" was a happy memory and Charles Busch, whose plays and performance had received favorable reviews, was an emblem of a quirky kind of acceptance of gay performance by a dominant culture. And it was an evening of funny entertainment and often riveting stage presence, made more extraordinary by the anniversary it marked as well as by the fact that the production took place not in some Village dive but at the mainstream Town Hall. At a time of struggle that has often been configured as war, such productions are at the very least "entertaining the troops."[45]

McCourt's high-culture allusions are in contrast with Tim Miller's pop-culture references to Denny's restaurants and to David Cassidy of TV's "The Partridge Family" or David Drake's references to middle-brow Broadway musicals *Pippin* and Bernstein's *West Side Story*. At first glance, these seem simply a difference in style. However, as Hodge and Kress point out, style isn't simple, but is rather a "metasign" that creates and sustains difference and identity.[46] In this case the densely allusive style of McCourt's writing, the high-culture domains of most of those references, and his virtuosic prose, signify a reading audience of the first generations of gay men just before and after Stonewall, whereas Miller's and Drake's styles, characterized by their mass-culture references and less dense prose structures, construct a performance audience of younger queer men, the second post-Stonewall generation. However, the distinction between "gay" and "queer" is predicated on more than a generational cohort. Not necessarily ideologically assimilationist, though perhaps more inclined toward external social conformity, "gay" implies an essentialist notion of sexuality and desire, and tacitly accepts the homo/hetero binarism. The postmodern "queer," however, connotes a social constructionist belief in the polymorphous nature of all sexuality and desire, and it deconstructs not only the binarism of homo/hetero but eventually male/female. Remaining unresolved, however, is the essentialist/constructionist binary opposition.[47] Typically, in the early 1980s faced with the initial depredations of AIDS, people of McCourt's generation would establish AIDS service organizations like New York's Gay Men's Health Crisis (GMHC), while people of Miller's and Drake's, faced with bureaucractic inertia and health politics, would establish the "Queer Nation" of the late 1980s and 1990s and would enlist in the ranks of ACT UP.

In *Time Remaining* McCourt plays with the modernist notion that, in myth, time past is also time present; and not only time past, but time future as well has a nostalgic quality, as though the future were also remembered:

> *Where does this difference between the past and the future come from? Why do we remember the past but not the future?*—you see, some do—and, *Why does disorder increase in the same direction of time as that in which the universe expands?* Which is the same as asking why do I get smarter as my body gets weaker, only to lose all my marbles in the end? (81)

This inquiry into entropy is one of numerous apocalyptic allusions in a book that Walter Kendrick has characterized as "suffused with what the professorial Bloom calls belatedness, the sense of having lived on into an age when everything that matters has already happened" and which carries "the grim knowledge that, as Tony Kushner's Broadway extravaganza proclaims, *Millennium Approaches*."[48] Is this the entropic fin de siècle or the millennialist apocalypse with its promise of marriage and rebirth? A bit of both, I think, since Odette in part registers the apocalypse as a memory, forestalls a cathartic cataclysm with camping irony, and rescripts the whole story at its Edenic origins:

> [I]f old Yeats were to be resurrected and come to New York, and attend an Ashbery reading, and read through the publicity handouts—all the awards, all the laurels rained down on the head—he would be absolutely convinced that Aleister Crowley had won the final day, that the Age of Pandemonium had indeed been inaugurated to run its full thousand-year term. . . . It's not as if we've had our last sentimental feeling image, our last regression, even if the word is out that everybody now ought to be consciously *post*-millenarian—which as one girl remarked when told of same, "Well, honey, they are right *on* about that, whoever said it; hardly anybody you know even *owns* a hat." But I think the most beautiful thing I heard the professor [Harold Bloom] say, practically off the cuff, about art and life and nostalgia—the best thing, really, I'd heard since Paris in the forties [sic]—was this: *Paradise is forever* there *and our knowing is* here, *but our being is split off from our knowing, and so it turns out that we still abide in Eden.* Wouldn't that just take your *breath* away? It did mine—for a whole day. (90–92)

In this last assertion, McCourt's Delancey resonates with Tim Miller's utopian refusal to leave Eden, but where Miller reveals his exposed naked queer body with its Adamically named parts, McCourt reveals only Odette (and to a lesser extent Delancey) revealing themselves. Since "apocalypse" derives from the Greek word for "revelation," such disclosures are to be expected. McCourt's writing is a drag, the *vesture* of language that even the *gesture* of the performance artist cannot strip away. His dedication of *Time Remaining*, "In memory of dead friends pictured within," and his characterization of the book as "an amalgamation of stories, schoolfriends, people from the line at the Met. Mainly it's about people from New York"[49] underscores the extent to which this book slides from documentary (Jackson Pollock is outed) to autobiography (references to *New Yorker* editor and Village habitué Dorothy Dean's witticisms) to roman á clef (poet James Schuyler as "The Skylark" or Holly Woodlawn as, well, "Holly Woodlawn"). While revealing Odette and Delancey, McCourt remains in authorial drag. Where Miller, and to a lesser extent Drake, reveal by stripping off, McCourt reveals by putting on; in this case the drag performance consists of written discourse.

In order to claim McCourt's written text as a drag performance, I want to invoke Roland Barthes' "Theory of the Text," particularly the performance and clothing tropes that illuminate my claims for McCourt's book. Toward the beginning of that essay, Barthes teases out the etymological implications of the word "text":

> Constitutively linked with writing (the text is *what is written*), perhaps because the very graphics of the letter—although remaining linear— suggest not speech, but the interweaving of a tissue (etymologically speaking, "text" means "tissue"), the text is, in the work, what secures the guarantee of the written object, bringing together its safe-guarding functions: on the one hand the stability and permanence of inscription, desiring to correct the fragility and imprecision of the memory, and on the other hand the legality of the letter, that incontrovertible and indelible trace, supposedly, of the meaning which the author has intentionally placed in his work; the text is a weapon against time, oblivion and the trickery of speech . . . [50]

The apocalyptic text attempts doubly so to be a "weapon against time [and] oblivion" in a way McCourt establishes by his interweaving of reminiscence and oracular utterance within Delancey's and Odette's conversation. And certainly the modernist claims of *Time Remaining*—not only the Joycean narration but also its (narrator's) mythic consciousness—situate the book as an effort to transcend time through a mythic essentialism. After all, Delancey recalls, "I remember *everybody* telling the *same* story over and over again. . . . Could be there's only ever been one story. (Tick-tock. This-that. Envelope structure and all.)" (66). However, Barthes contrasts this logocentrism with the poststructuralist theory of the text, which he characterizes as "hyphology":

> [Text] is a tissue, something woven. But whereas criticism (to date the only known form, in France, of a theory of literature) hitherto unanimously placed the emphasis on the finished "fabric" (the text being a "veil" behind which the truth, the real message, in a word the 'meaning,' had to be sought), the current theory of the text turns away from the text as veil and tries to perceive the fabric in its texture, in the interlacing of codes, formulae and signifiers, in the midst of which the subject places himself and is undone, like a spider that comes to dissolve itself into its own web. A lover of neologisms might therefore define the theory of the text as a "hyphology" ('hyphos' is the fabric, the veil . . .). [51]

To borrow from the title of James Purdy's AIDS fiction, words are "Garments the Living Wear"; and we are what we wear.

McCourt's Delancey does not pretend that the mythic text makes any transcendant sense:

> One thing I know, and that is that my telling the stories of the dead is in no way bringing order of any kind to a mass of experience the better to preserve it—or anything like that malarkey you still sometimes hear literary theorists peddle. I hold—as Odette would say—with the implications of the painting of Jackson Pollock, and with the ideas of the author of *A Brief History of Time*, the crippled English genius who seems to nearly know the secret of the universe, but who noted,
>
>> Thus the heat expelled by the computer's cooling fan means that when a computer records an item in memory, the total amount of disorder in the universe still goes up. (67)

Mythic performance seems more of a habit than anything else. And although Odette claims to be postmodern, even "post-*contemporary*," she seems almost fundamentalist in her zest for naturalistic signification:

> I don't myself go in for consciously hidden meanings at all. I like my meanings *manifest*, don't-cha know, the way I like my men: hung all over the place, and *bulging*, like the plumbing on the outside of the Beaubourg. All the same, dear, like any metaphor—like any *man*, too—it works best the first time you get it up. Later, even an afternoon later, there are bound to be . . . which doesn't mean you discard it, not necessarily. Only that you *note* diligently its deficiencies, and come to terms. Ditto fusion texts and holograms, cyberspace and autofellatio. (75)

As in Tim Miller's peroration to his penis—which linked its nonperformance in the erotic space with that of gay men in the political space—McCourt's Odette acknowledges the performative theatricality of the text, a point not far from Barthes' point when he characterizes a text as "the very theatre of a production where the producer and reader of the text meet." The performativity of the written or "fixed" text occurs when "the scriptor and/or the reader begin to play with the signifier."[52] *Time Remaining* travesties apocalyptic discourse's transcendental fictions—the desire to transcend time and entropy—but remains conscious of the drag. As Delancey, who has the book's first and last word, observes: "(For there is no question of life that is not fundamentally a question of death—*that* I know: that goes without saying, in spite of the fact that we can never stop talking about it.) I'd heard the bell: I had a performance to give" (68). Because talk is all we have, we all have to talk. Or as Odette might have said, without my meaning to put words in her mouth, *Je parle, donc je suis.*

American apocalypticism is ensnared in a performative contradiction. On the one hand, apocalyptic discourse presumes stable subjectivities (the elect/the damned; the clean/the unclean) whose binaries admit of no intervening registers; on the other hand, such putatively stable identities have been rehearsed, re-presented, reenacted, almost obssessively, certainly ritually, from the beginning of the European colonization of North America, so much so that apocalyptic performance seems America's hallmark ritual. While asserting its stability through essentialist binary categories, apocalyptic discourse betrays its very temporality and contingency: identity is not essential but performative, and subjectivity exists in the moment of performance, not as a stable text. Perhaps another way to put it: we *pretend* who we are. I have in mind a secondary significance of "pretend": to stretch forth, to project. As Tim Miller and David Román underscore "coming out" and "conversion" are not stable states, but entail "a lifelong project of continuous self-identification and revelations."[53] There is no end to the performance of subjectivity and for that very reason one does not "accomplish" it in any definitive or permanent way. Similarly, performances and texts produce in audiences and readers only transitory effects; their work, only provisional.

American apocalyptic rituals would seem to be our primary vehicles for the production of identity. In the United States we tend to construct our politics around crisis, war, and demons, mortared with a sense of mission. As Leon Festinger, Henry Riecken, and Stanley Schachter have pointed out, apocalyptic performances that posit a specific end time can be repeated, even after prophetic expectations have been disappointed, which indicates how little apocalypticism has to do with the closure of time and how much with the (desire for) closure of subjectivity. That desire sometimes leads to the catastrophic closures we have witnessed in Jonestown, Waco, and September 11.[54]

Tim Miller, David Drake, and James McCourt all employ a variation on the Puritan spiritual autobiography, with its components of "calling, conversion, temptation resisted, and regenerate living," a form that can only be understood from an apocalyptic perspective that endows history with a trajectory. All three performances that I have explored here participate in the discursive form that Bercovitch calls "auto-American-biography: the celebration of the representative self as America, and of

the American self as the embodiment of a prophetic universal design."
This form is characterized "not only [by] the persistent influence of
millennialism, but [by] the overall consistency of rhetoric and approach,"
a rhetoric that "survived, finally, not by chance but by merit, because it
was compelling enough in content and flexible enough in form to invite
adaptation." Probably the most central discursive ritual of North American gay people is the coming out story, narrating how one came to
acknowledge one's own queerness and began to perform or "pretend" it.
Ironically, this ritual is homologous to the evangelical's "born again"
conversion narrative, both in the sense that these narrative rituals construct an originary point (the conversion experience[s]) and in that their
repetition edifies individuals and collectives, shoring up the fragility of
the speaking subject and the listening audience. The American typological imagination allows the audience or reader to identify itself in the
representative performer or writer. The solo performance artist, like the
preacher or evangelical witness, becomes another "authorized version" of
individual and communal identity, even in relatively secular spaces like
the West Village's Perry Street Theater or the East Village's P.S. 122. As
Marvin Carlson points out, "This sense of providing a voice and body to
common (and generally unarticulated) experience is very important to
much modern performance, especially that created by and for marginalized
or oppressed communities" and although solo performance is "still built
upon the physical presence of the performer, [it] relies heavily upon the
word, and very often upon the word as revelation of the performer,
through the use of autobiographical material." The physical spaces themselves are contingent and provisional, because an elementary school can
become a performance venue, a police building can become a theater, or
a church can become a disco.[55]

Personalizing the apocalypse is thus not foreign to this discursive
field, especially in its American manifestations. The exilic messengers
preaching alarm and hope, like Miller, Drake, and McCourt, stand in for,
stand up for, and stand up to the audience addressed. In the next chapter,
I examine a related rhetorical structure, the prophetic jeremiad, and one
of its most persistent modern practitioners, the playwright, novelist, and
AIDS activist, Larry Kramer.

Chapter Three

Larry Kramer and the American Jeremiad

(In memory of Ray)

When his essay, "1,112 and Counting," first appeared in the March 14–27, 1983 issue of the *New York Native*, the city's premier gay newspaper with a largely male audience, Larry Kramer was continuing a venerable American discursive tradition. Its opening sentences evoked doom:

> If this article doesn't scare the shit out of you, we're in real trouble. If this article doesn't rouse you to anger, fury, rage, and action, gay men may have no future on this earth. Our continued existence depends on just how angry you can get.

Its conclusion called for volunteer action and civil disobedience. Kramer's essay represented an American genre typified by both lament and celebration: a warning about impending judgment combined with the hope of renewal and repair, the jeremiad sermon. Sacvan Bercovitch has characterized the American jeremiad as "a ritual designed to join social criticism to spiritual renewal, public to private identity, the shifting 'signs of the times' to certain traditional metaphors, themes, and symbols" that "persuades in proportion to its capacity to help people act in history." Perhaps no discursive form has been as pervasive in American culture as a means of composing communal identity, one that requires a community either to renew or to redefine its mission. We see the persistence of this rhetoric all around us in the language of the scolds who populate the American landscape today, from conservatives, on the one hand, who decry our decline into a welfare state while holding up the ideal of

63

American self-reliance, to the progressives, on the other hand, who decry a politics of self-interest while holding up an American tradition of solidarity.[1]

Before the first Puritan colonists landed on the shores of North America, their leader John Winthrop warned them that though they were God's faithful remnant they would nonetheless be dispossessed if they were not faithful to their Divine covenant. While Winthrop had reason for concern about that fragile community's survival when he sounded the note of doom and expectation as the *Arbella* came to shore, by the time of the Colonial period a pattern of American discourse was fixed in the form we read and hear today:

> No doubt [Winthrop's] threats were prompted in part by anxiety; their very stridency speaks of hardships to come in settling an unknown land. But more significant . . . is how closely they foreshadow the major themes of the colonial pulpit. False dealing with God, betrayal of covenant promises, the degeneracy of the young, the lure of profits and pleasures, the prospect of God's just, swift, and total revenge—it reads like an index of favorite sermon topics of seventeenth-century New England. In particular . . . the political sermon—what might be called the state-of-the-covenant address, tendered at every public occasion . . . which has been designated as the jeremiad.

One does not need to have been religious to have heard the jeremiad, a form employed with equal effect by American preachers, politicians, and secular social critics.[2]

As a species of prophetic utterance, the jeremiad is arguably not an apocalyptic genre. Apocalypse, after all, assumes the existence of a universal principle of evil pitted against a universal principle of good, rather than human resistance to divine good. These two forces are poised for ultimate battle in which humans are swept up. In addition, apocalypse views human agency as limited to patient endurance, whereas the prophetic jeremiad is precisely a call for conversion, decisive human action. In apocalypse, catastrophe cannot be avoided; in prophetic utterance, repentance prevents the wrath of God. These distinctions, however, are largely academic in the context of this study. Biblical scholars can valuably distinguish between earlier prophetic and later apocalyptic discourses in the canon of Hebrew scriptures, but the culture criticism that I am performing here insists on examining the cultural work these utterances perform, not the theological or philosophical distinctions that they make regarding human freedom. Both apocalyptic and prophetic doom utterances normalize crisis and precipitate group solidarity in much the same way.[3]

I argue that Larry Kramer's high-profile AIDS activism reproduced the discursive tradition of the jeremiad and relied on its rhetorical effects. In particular, his earlier pre-AIDS writing, especially the controversial 1978 novel *Faggots*, is jeremiadic and to a great extent his discourse relies on the "static oppositions" and the normalizing of crisis that typify the jeremiad. Kramer's later plays, essays, letters to the editor, and speeches all tended to rely on sharp binary oppositions and an intensified sense of urgency, both of which made him by the early 1990s America's most outspoken and effective AIDS activist as well as one of the most resented or, worse, ignored.[4]

NORMALIZING CRISIS

Sacvan Bercovitch observes of the American jeremiad, distinct from its European forms, that "[i]t made anxiety its end as well as its means. Crisis was the social norm it sought to inculcate. . . . New England's Jeremiahs set out to provide the sense of insecurity that would ensure the outcome. Denouncing or affirming, their vision fed on the distance between promise and fact."[5] Perhaps because of Americans' tremendous appetite for distraction and the extensive late-capitalist resources employed simultaneously to relieve and to stimulate that hunger, we only pay attention to social concerns when they are presented as crises. What precisely constitutes a "crisis" is elusive since the term is more than most a rhetorical trope intended to mobilize action, a marketing tactic in both the consumer market and in its counterpart in what passes as politics in the United States. In most discursive fields in the United States "consumers" or "citizens" only pay attention when addressed by someone invoking "crisis" even if only implicitly. News media use the term freely, in part to sell their products, "news stories," which are increasingly simply an extension of or pretext for the goods and services marketed by the sponsors who fund the media. Thus in a sense, news stories are marketing tools to get viewers or readers to attend to the real "story": consumer advertising.

An analysis of the relationship between "news" broadcasting/publication and advertisement broadcasting/publication is critical to the discursive context in which Larry Kramer found himself when he and others recognized the first outlines of a medical threat to their health and lives. New

York City is an enormous market for products and services and therefore a huge media market, both locally and nationally. In the first years of the AIDS epidemic, extensive and front-page coverage—the kind that gets people's attention and prompts a response—was relegated to the *New York Native* while the frequency and significance of reports in the *New York Times* were few and small. The semiotic fields of New York are so densely overgrown that the only signs that get read are those that are large or loud, and repeated. Newspapers, for example, feature full-page advertisements for movies. Tabloid papers like the *News* or *Newsday* sport large-type headlines regardless of an event's significance. Buildings' empty walls and construction partitions are plastered with wheat-pasted bills, the same bill repeated many times in many rows. Human-size billboards in subways and gargantuan ones on Times Square compete for pedestrians' attention.

Apocalypticism's sense of crisis, itself the product of a binary opposition composed of safety/danger or rescue/catastrophe, is particularly suited to the post-print world of profusely reproduced and competing signs, the modern and postmodern worlds since the sixteenth century, which also marks, not coincidentally I think, the emergence of Protestant apocalypticism. In "Criticism as Activism" James Miller problematizes the term "crisis," by noting its history in English from its mid-sixteenth-century neologistic entry as a medical term (which had shifted from an earlier significance as a juridical term), to its use in fields of history, politics, and spirituality during the English Civil War of the seventeenth century, and its eventual deployment in the nineteenth century as a literary critical term applied to drama. This lexical genealogy presents several different "narratives" that may be composed around a point of "crisis":

> What sort of crisis, then, is the "the [sic] AIDS crisis"? That would seem to depend not wholly on the biological peculiarities of the syndrome itself or on the relentless spread of HIV from this population to that, as one might at first suppose. Rather, given the long evolution of "crisis mentality" in the West as a perceptual habit designed to organize events into a decisive plot, one can only conclude that it largely depends on certain cultural (that is, political, economic, religious, and even aesthetic) factors that have little to do with the "real world" of infected cells . . . and a great deal to do with the fantasy world of social agendas and conflicting discourses. What sort of AIDS crisis you find yourself in depends, then, on who constructs the narrative around the imagined turning-point, what sort of narrative is constructed, and why such construction is formed at such a time in such a place.

"Crisis" seems to enter the vacuum produced by the partial or full displacement of authority. As John Nguyet Erni contends:

> [T]he so-called AIDS crisis was in part *produced* as a focal point for the attempt to relegitimize organized, institutional, and technological medicine in a society that had grown skeptical of it prior to AIDS. All of this is part of the discourse of curing AIDS. All of it requires an explanation and analysis beyond the specific struggles of AIDS treatment. All of it suggests that the pair of contradictory discourses of AIDS has something to do with the crises and management of hegemony.

Kramer's crisis discourse, for example, is situated in the context of his struggle with and for authority both within the gay male community and within the professional medical bureaucracy. Furthermore, one of the difficulties of the AIDS epidemic has been that it is virtually impossible for individuals or collectives to maintain for very long a crisis ethos. Invariably one bureaucratizes the crisis (as with Gay Mens' Health Crisis, the first organization that Larry Kramer helped found) or exhausts one's resources and people (as with AIDS Coalition to Unleash Power, the second organization he helped found). American audiences tire of the same "crisis" or of the same approach to it and bestow their most stinging critique: they stop paying attention to the crisis, its prophets, and their message.[6]

KRAMER'S *FAGGOTS*

By the end of the 1970s many gay men in urban areas like New York and San Francisco had developed a complex culture constructed around desire and pleasure, establishing the gay "clone" as an urban type: instead of the stereotype of the effeminate queen, many post-Stonewall gay men reinvented themselves as hyper-masculine, dressed in uniforms of macho careers like police, cowboys, and construction workers, invented a social life that revolved around the disco, parties, gay resorts, and sexual adventures constituting "The Circuit" of New York. Since the 1950s and 1960s American attitudes had softened toward erotic and pharmaceutical ecstasies, so that the clone culture of the 1970s defined itself in part by its enjoyment of recreational sex and drugs, both of which seemed readily available, at least for those with either the economic or aesthetic capital to afford them. Among the assets of this culture were its democratizing of sexual relations across lines of class and career status and its network of friendships or families of affiliation that would in the earliest days of the AIDS epidemic produce an invaluable support network for gay men, many of whom had become estranged from their families of birth.[7]

Nonetheless, this urban culture was not without its deficits. Less physically attractive people had less aesthetic capital to barter for sex or status (which were sometimes indistinguishable). Class and race divisions might be abrogated on a case-by-case basis for a physically endowed man—or they might not or not for long. The clones' pursuit of pleasure seemed to some critics to have turned on them, requiring new stimulations for jaded tastes and leaving some observers with the suspicion that the pursuit may have been a flight from interpersonal psychosocial issues. To some commentators within the urban gay male communities many of these pleasures had become epidemics of substance abuse and sexually transmitted infections, not to mention short-lived intimate relationships. Although clone culture had emerged from notions of radical gay liberation, it was characteristically apolitical:

> Like many others, when Gay Pride marches started down Fifth Avenue at the end of June, I was on Fire Island. Gay politics had an awful image. Loudmouths, the unkempt, the dirty and unwashed, men in leather or dresses, fat women with greasy slicked-back ducktail hairdos. Another world. Certainly not a world that connected with mine. Nor did I want it to. On Fire Island, we laughed, in those long-ago days of health, when we watched the evening news on Sunday night flash brief seconds of those straggling, pitiful marches.[8]

It was in this context that Larry Kramer published his novel, *Faggots* in 1978. Intending a satire of urban gay life with Evelyn Waugh's novels of social satire as his model, Kramer discovered that in some gay political circles his critique of clone culture was unwelcome and was greeted with hostility. In an op-ed piece for the *New York Times* shortly after the novel's publication, Kramer compared the warmth, activism, and sense of community he had recently experienced in San Francisco at a memorial for slain activist and politician, Harvey Milk, to the gays of his own home town: "I am back in New York, missing, very much, the sense of community I felt in San Francisco. I call several of my friends, but no one is home. I know that most of my friends are at the bars or the baths or the discos, tripping out on trivia."[9]

Despite a mixed critical reception upon publication in 1978, *Faggots* has gone on to be a best-selling novel, reissued in 1987. James Miller suggests that some of the outrage among gay readers of the novel resulted from the fact that:

> Consciences were pricked. Pricks were exposed to the anaphrodisiac strokes of conscience (colder by far than the fingers of the sea). No televangelist in the service of the Heterosexist Panopticon could have poured a colder shower on the boys in the sand than an informed source like Kramer—a dancer from their own dance. Much to their embarrassed surprise, he was utterly serious in his condemnation of their "Beatific Vision" as a glamorous illusion, a trashing of the high ideals of Gay Culture in a Gehenna of lost souls.

In a careful study of Kramer's rhetoric from his screenplay for the film version of D. H. Lawrence's *Women in Love* to his AIDS activism today, David Bergman distinguishes Kramer's treatment of "The Circuit" with that of Andrew Holleran's *Dancer from the Dance* and Edmund White's *Nocturnes for the King of Naples* (all published the same year):

> What separates White and Holleran from Kramer and what freed them from an angry backlash is that they possess a lyric sympathy for their wayward characters, while Kramer, at best, musters an angry identification. Unlike Evelyn Waugh, Kramer's artistic model, Kramer never gained the requisite distance or clinical detachment. His personal involvement interferes with both his sympathy and objectivity. Where White and Holleran are sweetly elegiac, Kramer is bitterly censorious.

Those features continue to characterize much of their writing even today. In her review for the *Washington Post*, Barbara Harrison worried that *Faggots* would only give Anita Bryant and her comrades more ammunition. Martin Duberman, former director of the Center for Lesbian and Gay Studies at City University of New York, characterized the book as "foolish . . . stupid" precisely because it failed as a satire of the Fire Island clone culture:

> I say this as someone who can't stand the place, who thinks it magnifies the worst aspects of gay male life and lends credence to the standard homophobic equation of gayness with narcissism and mindlessness. A serious dissection of the self-absorbed frivolity of this subculture within a subculture would be well worth having. But it would have to be one capable of seeing that "obsessive triviality" does not encompass the reality of a style whose exuberant, risky raunchiness we may one day

realize contained the seeds of a far-reaching social transformation. *Faggots* is not remotely that needed dissection. It is a plastic, trashy artifact of the worst aspects of a scene to which it high-mindedly condescends.

Kramer was both explicit in his narrative description and unrelenting in his contempt, an approach that would also come to characterize his AIDS activism.[10]

In *Faggots'* third-person narration, Kramer recounts the quest of gay urbanite, writer Fred Lemish, as he seeks a loving, stable relationship moving among the worlds of business, Manhattan discotheques and sex clubs, and Fire Island cottages and dunes. The object of Fred Lemish's affections is Dinky Adams, whom Lemish and the novel follow from one sexual adventure to another, culminating in a Fire Island dune orgy. The novel is unified around this quest, which is introduced at its beginning: "Had he not decided to write about a Voyage of Discovery into this World in which he lived? This Faggot World"[11] and continued to its last episode: "OK, Lemish. Your journey now begins. Your work is now cut out for you. Your hard work. From this moment not one other opinion matters but your own. There will always be enemies. Time to stop being your own" (300). This gay Adam prepares to expel himself from the erotic Garden of Eden. At first Lemish thinks his quest is for the elusive Dinky, who is characterized as a Holy Grail in leather pants (262). Additionally, in a critique of pharmacological ecstasies (and of the predatory and Wagnerian character, The Gnome, a drug dealer), Kramer writes: "Fred took no drugs. He'd tried them all, found no answers, and he was on a pilgrimage for answers" (121). Like Parsifal's, the quest entails questions. One question posed by self-described agnostic Kramer early in the novel is "The straight and narrow, so beloved of our founding fathers and all fathers, is now obviously and irrevocably bent. What is God trying to tell us . . . ?" (3–4). Another question, posed by the pseudonymous columnist "Blaze Sorority," would become one of Kramer's significant laments in the 1980s: "And now, brothers and sisters, let me be sad. Let me be. Oh, my little babies, where is he? Where oh where oh where? And when he appears, will we know him? Will we follow him? Will we love, respect, admire, emulate, follow him? Oh Miss God: Give us a leader to follow. A Hero!" (87). Overwhelmed by the frantic energy of a Fire Island disco dance floor, a minor character, Josie, shouts over the music to Fred, " 'Summer after summer. Another repetition of a repetition. Weekends without number. All the same thing. Starting up all over again.

Do I have the courage to leave it? Go somewhere? Go to where? To do what? So much energy. So much. Why leave it? Why stay? So much. Toward what end?' " (297). Often self-consciously, the novel attempts to recommend answers to some of those questions.

In the closing episode of the novel, which takes place in a patch of island woods dubbed The Meat Rack, Fred Lemish observes Dinky being "fisted": "Dinky just continued to jerk up in pleasure and smile at heaven. That elusive heaven. Now so close. Now almost here. [Dinky] tried to say a few more words . . . 'I . . . I . . . I . . . want . . . your . . . other . . . arm!" (283). In this voyeuristic moment Lemish has a Joycean epiphany: "Fred looks at all and thinks immortal thoughts, not of Adams, Dinky, for a change, but of Miller, Henry: 'We are no longer animals but we are certainly not yet men.' Which happily at last gives him a tidge of courage to think heroic thoughts of Lemish, Fred: 'The fucking we're getting's not worth the fucking we're getting,' and it's time to go . . . So, feeling that the now discovered smithy of his sex appears no longer worth the forag-ing [sic], he bends to kiss his Dinky 'Bye' and he turns to leave" (285). This epiphany renders Lemish a "phoenix from the ashes" as he comes to a "New Era, A.D., After Dinky" (292). Sometimes this discourse is explicitly apocalyptic, as when the hysterical crowd gathering for the opening of a new club is compared to *Day of the Locust* (173) or when in one Fire Island party scene, Fred replies to the question, "What is happening to us?" with the pronouncement, "We're all going crazy. We're out of control. I think it's the end of the world" (235).

In reading *Faggots* back through the filter of the AIDS epidemic, we can find Kramer's apparent prescience sometimes eerie. His alter ego, Lemish, obsesses about his body. For example, when Lemish goes to the bathroom (a frequent concern of this character):

> He noted that the shit was falling in squiggles and this caused him, naturally, to be fearful. Had he once again come down with a case of last year's fashionable disease, the galloping trots, known medically as amebiasis, an amebic dysentery, also known in the gay world as the P.R. disease, there being a good deal of it around ("of epidemic propor-tions," Fred finally discovered from a Dr. Kelvin Knell)? Fred had caught it, not from foreign travel, but, so far as Mini Diary calculations could reveal, at the Everhard [bathhouse]. (91)

However, before attributing Kramer with a super- or at least preternatural foresight, one should remember that physicians with a sexually-active, urban gay male clientele had become concerned about the rates and types of sexually transmitted diseases found in some of their patients, a public health fact that religious and political conservatives would exploit after the appearance of AIDS.[12]

KRAMER'S AIDS ACTIVISM

From 1981, the year AIDS entered public discourse in New York City and elsewhere, Larry Kramer would become a vocal activist on behalf of the sick and the HIV infected, in addition to the larger gay and lesbian community. This activism took a variety of forms: letters to the editor of local and national newspapers and magazines, op-ed essays and articles, plays, and speeches, a discursive flood proportional to that arising from the epidemic generally. In an appeal to New York's gay men appearing in the August 24–September 6, 1981 issue of *New York Native*, at the time the city's newest gay paper, only four months after Dr. Lawrence Mass' first article appeared in the same periodical and two months after Lawrence Altman's in the *Times*, Kramer urged financial support for treatment of Kaposi's sarcoma patients. He admonished the readers: "This is our disease and we must take care of each other and ourselves. In the past we have often been a divided community; I hope we can all get together on this emergency, undivided, cohesively, and with all the numbers we in so many ways possess."[13]

But Kramer's suggestion of an epidemiology for the cancer, backgrounded by his earlier critique of urban gay clone culture and its excesses, would make Kramer the target of criticism by other gay men:

> The men who have been stricken don't appear to have done anything that many New York gay men haven't done at one time or another. We're appalled that this is happening to them and terrified that it could happen to us. It's easy to become frightened that one of the many things we've done or taken over the past years may be all that it takes for a cancer to grow from a tiny something-or-other that got in there who knows when from doing who knows what.

What seems now to us like a benign epidemiological speculation informed by the growing popular understanding of the environmental causes of illness, struck writer Robert Chesley rather differently in a response to Kramer's appeal three issues later:

Basically, Kramer *is* telling us that something we gay men are doing (drugs? kinky sex?) is causing Kaposi's sarcoma. . . . But there's another issue here. It is always instructive to look closely at emotionalism, for it so often has a hidden message which is the *real* secret of its appeal. I think the concealed meaning in Kramer's emotionalism is the triumph of guilt: that gay men *deserve* to die for their promiscuity. In his novel *Faggots*, Kramer told us that sex is dirty and that we ought not to be doing what we're doing. Now, with Kaposi's sarcoma attacking gay men, Kramer assumes he knows the cause . . . and—well, let's say that it's easy to become frightened that Kramer's *real* emotion is a sense of having been vindicated, though tragically: he told us so, but we didn't listen to him, sooo—we had to learn the hard way, and now we're dying.[14]

Chesley's own rhetorical excesses here signify something of his own emotional landscape at the time, and five issues later (in late December 1981) Kramer replied in characteristically personal terms to Chesley and others who had responded that autumn:

Bob has not been completely honest with either *Native* readers or his political constituency. We had been friends, and I find it curious that his attacks upon me in print commenced with the cessation of this relationship. From the reporter who arrived at my apartment as a "fan," quoting to me his favorite lines from *Faggots*, effusive in his admiration for it, he turned, rather suddenly I thought, into someone who has been attacking me in print ever since. His list of my malfeasances is endless. He has already trotted out homophobia, anti-eroticism, self-loathing, sex-as-evil, Anita Bryantism, brainwashed-by-psychoanalysis, fascism.[15]

Of course, Chesley had not explicitly made those claims in his letter, but the discourse of both writers had escalated accordingly.

In his response, however, Kramer had an opportunity to clarify what I think for him have been dominant themes in his modern jeremiads:

In *Faggots*, I set out to try to understand one main issue: why did I see so little love between two homosexual men? Love is what I wanted and want, and what most of the friends I have say they want, too. . . . What does it take for all of us to work together? Why is Bob Chesley attacking *me*? Why is he not attacking the CDC for taking so long to prepare their epidemiological studies? Why is he not attacking the National Cancer Institute and the American Cancer Society . . . ? Why is Bob Chesley attacking me? Why is he not asking every homosexual in this

city: Why are we here? What are we here for?. . . What is this dream
world we inhabit? Why is our community so impotent and lethargic?
Is everything *too* good for us? Do we need Dunkirks before we can
organize and fight back? Until then, can we only hurt each other?[16]

Stable relationships, gay unity, and a sense of purpose or mission were
Kramer's central moral concerns in the attempt to articulate an ideal
social and political queer community, one that starts with the individual
and expands to couples and other larger gay collectives.

Not all the responses to Kramer's earliest AIDS writing were as suspicious as Chesley's. Arthur Bell noted his dislike for what he perceived
as Kramer's erotophobia in *Faggots*, but acknowledged that Kramer was
"the force that got together a number of people who are organizing
support groups for those victims of the 'gay cancer,' and finding ways and
means of funding research into the cancer that's zeroed in on over a
hundred of us. Larry's efforts are sincere to the point of being almost
zealot-like and he should be applauded, really applauded." In that same
issue of the *Native*, Nathan Fain wrote to criticize Chesley's "attack" on
Kramer, characterizing it as reflecting "the moral posture of an iguana"
(an analogy that is not utterly clear; perhaps he meant "chameleon"),
defending Kramer's novel and characterizing Chesley as a "cruel faggot"
who deserved a special place in hell. In a later issue of the paper, Scott
Tucker in Philadelphia defended Chesley's suspicions about *Faggots* (which
he had reviewed and panned) while admiring and supporting Kramer's
call to action.[17]

After Kramer's response appeared during the winter holidays, several
ripostes appeared in the first issue of 1982. Robert Chesley acknowledged
that he was a "rejected trick" of Kramer, but repudiated Kramer's implication that the erotic failure motivated Chesley's criticism; in addition, he
articulated the critical differences he had with Kramer:

> [H]e is the most prominent and clearest exponent of certain (usually)
> unconscious strains of thought and/or feeling in gay life and literature
> that I find pernicious and that I hope gay people will think about.
> These are: 1) anti-eroticism; 2) guilt and the desire for punishment;
> and 3) moralism and the adulation of authority.

Owen Wilson, writing in the same issue, condemned Kramer's use of
guilt tactics and suggested that "[t]he point is that gay guys are dying and
we damn well better find out why. Period. Kramer will raise more money

and more support if he stops calling us names and laying guilt trips on us." A third letter came from a writer signing himself as "Francis Xavier Boynton, Jr." who parodied the personal invective of the correspondence to date.[18]

In that same issue, Kramer had the opportunity to respond to each, though most of his fire (and ire) was directed toward Chesley, of whom Kramer wondered, "Why do Chesley's demons smack so of religion?" Kramer articulated his dissent from the sexual dissidents asserting, "Yes, I think that people should not fuck in the IRT or the streets. . . . It's almost laughable that this is being used as a charge against me. If this is all we stand for, no wonder the City Council scorns us and the Mayor refuses to participate in our activities on Gay Liberation Day. How long must we remain so small-minded and reductionist that we are still fighting for the right to be judged solely by our sexual appetites?" In concluding his response, Kramer again articulated his vision of gay community: "Perhaps because I am one, I always expect homosexuals to be better than other people."[19]

In the following issue of the newspaper, several respondents continued the conversation, mostly in support of Kramer. Richard Umans applauded Kramer's leadership on the Kaposi's sarcoma crisis, but denounced his "whiny, self-serving, and tasteless defenses of himself and his literary standing." Gay activist Arnie Kantrowitz decried the personal dimensions of the Kramer-Chesley correspondence, but affirmed Kramer's message and asserted that "there's a more important issue here: survival . . . to keep as many faggots alive as possible, for both personal and political reasons." Richard Haber's letter applauded Kramer without reservation: "Bravo Larry Kramer! He is standing up for what is positive and responsible in gay life by recognizing and identifying what is destructive and self-defeating."[20]

In the first issue of February, whose characteristically sensational cover headline on a double murder announced "Gay Men Executed in Village," the correspondence continued. Writing in defense of Kramer, Michael Hirsch noted that "we are creating a community of separateness by our communal and individual actions, and by closing ourselves off we cause the ultimate harm to ourselves." Hirsch's letter also claimed that the gay male community was continuing "to disregard such things as personal hygiene and communal social responsibilities" and proposed an assimilationist agenda: "In seeking acceptance, respect, and our civil rights from other members of society, we should accept or at least use some of the ground rules that they live their lives by." Edward Sherman took a more satirical or camp view of the Kramer-Chesley correspondence: "There is no truth to the rumor that Bette Davis has been signed to play the role of Larry Kramer in the film version of 'Letters to the Editor.' Nor is there any truth to the rumor that the Brothers Warner are searching frantically for a 'Robert Chesley' type—now that Miriam Hopkins is dead." Finally, the controversy exhausted itself momentarily in the second February 1982 issue with two letters critical of Kramer. Robert Cromwell characterized Kramer as a "puritan [sic] letting rip" and concluded that "Kramer's moral indignation is misplaced. He should save his wrath for those he's beginning to sound like, the so-called Moral Majority." Pete Wilson asserted that by condoning police arrests of men having sex in subway toilets Kramer "aligns himself with fag-haters and queer bashers."[21]

Several things seem remarkable to me about this earliest entry of Larry Kramer's AIDS activist discourse. First, the exchange, particularly the Kramer-Chesley correspondence, offers a different spin on the feminist axiom that "the personal is the political." Despite New York City's claims as a massive metropolitan center, the gay male community, especially among its culture workers and among those living in and around Greenwich Village (including the East Village and, to the north, Chelsea) had constructed a dense network of relationships by turns professional, social, and erotic. As Kramer himself has pointed out:

> Because gays live in a ghetto, we know personally and generally recognize most of the people in it. We live together in this world-within-a-world: certain neighborhoods in Manhattan, Fire Island, the Hamptons; the discos we once danced in; the organizations we belong to . . [including] AIDS organizations in which we attempt to take care of our own; or just walking down city streets everywhere. But even in rural areas of New York State and New Jersey and Staten Island, gays know where other gays are. It's like the old American idea of life in a small town. We know everybody.[22]

It might also be fair to offer a corollary to the axiom: "The *personality* is the political." The language of Kramer's AIDS activism even in this first year (as well as that of his respondents) was always already personal insofar as it signified not only his own ethical positions (e.g., sacrificing personal pleasure for a greater communal good) and embraced space normally categorized as "private," but also represented his complex subject positions as an erotic, desiring man, as a post-Holocaust American secular Jew, and as an increasingly visible member of a sexual minority community in an emerging identity politics, among others. Second, this discursive field seems to have been constructed from its first appearance within a regime shaped by oppositions. Out of Kramer's (to my mind) innocuous and cautious appeal for donations to help patients with Kaposi's sarcoma, Chesley responded with a dialectical antithesis based on his reading of Kramer, to which Kramer then responded in kind. Each letter to the editor by these two was simply the pretext for the next response onto which other themes were projected or in which each defined himself adversarially with regard to the other. Third, Kramer had announced his most basic positions, focusing on his expectations of personal and collective "responsibility," identity, and solidarity, within the first year of his emergence as an AIDS activist. It is clear, as Arthur Bell's letter in the October 19–November 1, 1981 issue of *New York Native* points out, that Kramer's vehemence concerning the so-called gay cancer was "zealot-like."

Finally, the sheer duration of the discussion is remarkable, even given the fact that the *New York Native* published every two weeks thus causing a delay in some writers' replies. Kramer's first published appeal for donations appeared in the August 24–September 6, 1981 issue and the publisher, Charles Ortleb, and editor, Tom Steele, continued printing responses through the February 15–28, 1982 issue, six months later. This discursive response hints at the intensity of other discussions not appearing in print, the emotional intensity with which those conversations were conducted, and the struggle over the power of self-representation of a "gay" identity.

APOCALYPTIC BINARISMS

In his satirical novel, *Faggots*, Kramer's announced aim was to provide a social criticism of urban and affluent gay culture. But as some readers pointed out, the novel's brittleness tended to present its characters, even its leading character, unsympathetically. With the inauguration of his AIDS activism, Kramer would continue to follow a pattern in which the rhetoric of idealism would become distorted by the rhetoric of disappointment, producing heroes who become demons or sometimes vice versa.

Two instances are illustrative. Kramer helped found two major AIDS organizations: New York's Gay Men's Health Crisis (GMHC) in 1981 and the direct action grassroots group, AIDS Coalition to Unleash Power (ACT UP) in 1987. In both cases, Kramer eventually turned against those organizations and their leadership when he became disappointed in the direction they had taken. In large measure, in fact, his call for an organization that would eventually become ACT UP arose from Kramer's disappointment with GMHC. Within two years of its founding, Kramer found himself marginalized from the board and leadership of GMHC, an alienation that would prompt him to become involved with the alternative AIDS Network. By 1985, when he took time away from the city in order to write his play, *The Normal Heart*, Kramer's disappointment with GMHC had become public in a series of articles critical of the organization he had founded, culminating in "open letters" to GMHC Executive Director Richard Dunne and Tim Sweeney, Deputy Director for Policy, published in *New York Native*. The letter to Dunne, appearing on January 26, 1987 lamented:

> I cannot for the life of me understand how the organization I helped to form has become such a bastion of conservativism and such a bureaucratic mess. The bigger you get, the more cowardly you become; the more money you receive, the more self-satisfied you are. No longer do you fight for the living; you have become a funeral home. You and your huge assortment of caretakers perform miraculous tasks helping the dying to die.

The letter to Sweeney, identifying Kramer's demands to reform the agency, followed in the next month. But a month later, at a March 10 meeting at the Gay and Lesbian Community Services Center in Greenwich Village, Kramer called for a new organization that would resume the course of direct action for which he thought GMHC had been founded and from which he believed it had strayed:

> But we desperately need leadership in this crisis. We desperately need a central voice and a central organization to which everything else can plug in and be coordinated through. There isn't anyone else. And in this area of centralized leadership, of vision, of seeing the larger picture and acting upon it, GMHC is tragically weak. It seems to have lost the sense of mission and urgency upon which it was founded.

The result in the weeks to follow was the formation of ACT UP.[23]

Two years after its founding, Kramer in a letter from the floor of its weekly meeting of November 27, 1989 would say, "Personally, ACT UP gives me my greatest energy and my greatest reason for being alive. We have already proved so much to the world and to our fellow gay men and lesbians." In a column in the *Newspaper of ACT UP* that fall Kramer would assert, "ACT UP is the most moving organization I have ever belonged to. And, week after week, one of the most moving experiences I have ever had in my life." However, in another "letter to the floor" of ACT UP on April 16, 1990, Kramer would charge, "I think we are turning rotten at our core. I think we are hitting out at each other more and more blindly and turning each other into the enemy." He would also characterize frustration among fellow activists as "something spreading around like the virus itself." More than a year later, at a speech he gave on the tenth anniversary of GMHC, Kramer would lament, "I look at the two organizations I helped to start, GMHC and ACT UP—my children—and I ask myself: What have we accomplished? And I am forced to answer: Very little." Among the objects of Kramer's angry disappointment was Dr. Suzanne Phillips, MD, a member of ACT UP who noted that in Kramer's estimation she had "gone from being a 'hero of the epidemic' to a 'hate-spewing viper,' all in a couple of months," and told Kramer, "You appear to be a person of extremes."[24]

Kramer painted individuals with whom he had been disappointed in the most categorical terms, as in the case of AIDS researcher and director of the National Institute for Allergy and Infectious Diseases (NIAID) of the National Institutes of Health (NIH), Dr. Anthony Fauci, who for Kramer has been either monster or savior. In an article for *New York Newsday* in May 1987, Kramer described Fauci as "being asked to do more than any human is capable of doing, with predictably human results. . . . Instead of screaming and yelling for help as loudly as he can, he tries to make do, to negotiate quietly." Later the next month, in a speech given in Boston to kick off that community's Gay and Lesbian Pride Week, Kramer characterized Fauci as "certainly not the enemy. Because he is not, and because I think he does care, I am even more angry at him for what he is not doing—no matter what his excuses, and he has many." What Fauci was not doing, in Kramer's analysis, was making as much noise as Kramer, resulting in funding going unused. Kramer acknowledged his own erotic attraction toward Fauci: "He's real cute. He's an Italian from Brooklyn, short, slim, compact; he wears aviator glasses and is a natty dresser, a very energetic and dynamic man" but undercut this description by noting, "Everybody likes Dr. Fauci and everybody thinks Dr. Fauci is real cute and every scientific person I spoke to whispers off to the side, 'Yes, he's real cute, but he's in way over his head.' " Testifying before the Reagan Presidential AIDS Commission in September 1987, Kramer again characterized Fauci as "way over his head" and accused him of mismanaging the AIDS Treatment Evaluation Units that he had organized.[25]

But Kramer employed his strongest invective in an "open letter" to Fauci published in the *Village Voice* in May, 1988: "I have been screaming at the National Institutes of Health since I first visited your Animal House of Horrors in 1984. I called you monsters then and I called you idiots in my play *The Normal Heart* and now I call you murderers." In this letter Kramer characterized Fauci as "an incompetent idiot" accusing him of mismanaging trials of drugs whose efficacy was promising. Further, Kramer suggested that Fauci was a "good lieutenant, like Adolf Eichmann" and repudiated the good intentions he had attributed to the scientist earlier: "You care, I'm told (although I no longer believe it). I've even heard you called a saint. You are in essence a scientist who's expected to be Lee Iacocca. But saints, miracle workers, good administrators, and brilliant scientists have imaginations vivid enough to know how to spend $374 million in a time of dire emergency. You have no imagination. You are banal (a word used so accurately to describe Eichmann)."[26]

The last reference, of course, was to Hannah Arendt's characterization of the "banality of evil" in *Eichmann in Jerusalem*. Arendt was one of several thinkers whom Kramer read in order to prepare a long essay, "Report from the Holocaust," for the first edition of his collected articles, speeches, and letters to the editor, and in which he drew explicit parallels between the AIDS crisis and the Nazi's "Final Solution." For Kramer, Fauci was an example of the federal government's "heinous . . . malfeasance" and along with President Reagan and other federal bureaucrats was "equal to Hitler and his Nazi doctors performing their murderous experiments in the camps—not because of similar intentions, but because of similar results."[27]

However, Kramer was also able to give Fauci credit where it was due. In an introductory essay, "Toward a Definition of Evil: Further Reports," prepared for the 1994 revised edition of his collected AIDS writings, Kramer noted that Fauci, "the government's chief point man on AIDS and, up to that moment, just about Number One on all our Public Enemies lists" had reversed his earlier resistance to changing drug testing protocols. Kramer's praise, though, is not without regret since the warming of relations between Fauci and activists like those of ACT-UP produced the bureaucratization of the activists rather than the radicalization of the bureaucrats. Likewise, for Kramer, a developing friendship with

Fauci complicated the rhetorical posture he had previously been able to strike:

> Before I knew him personally, it was in no way difficult for me to come after him like a maniacal tiger. As I came to know him over the following years (now that I'm HIV positive, he's even one of my doctors), even though I'm just as furiously angry at him for what he does and doesn't do, it's become painful for me to call him names. When I do criticize him in print, I find myself hoping he doesn't see the piece. He's a nice man with a lovely wife and he works seven days a week and rarely sees his kids. I have to remind myself that my idol Hannah Arendt pointed out for us all how nice people can perform so many evil deeds.[28]

These instances suggest something of the hegemonic power of dominant discourses, in which activists are bureaucratized and binary oppositions like "hero/demon" or "insider/outsider" are produced. As "outsiders," activists could employ the aggressively confrontational language of binary oppositions; however, once reconfigured as "insiders," they found themselves, in a sense, at a loss for words, eventually appropriating the language of liberal consensus in order to maintain their new status. Paradoxically, the oppositional discourse that might have sometimes "bought" activists' way into the inner circles, usually did not "pay their dues" to keep them there, which required another discursive habitus. In Kramer's case, for example, New York's Mayor Ed Koch refused to deal with the activist face to face precisely because of his oppositional discourse, though that same discursive form may eventually have secured Kramer's entré into the circles of national power with people like Anthony Fauci, especially after the success of his plays and the visibility of his articles and essays.

Kramer's "romance" with Fauci was evident in his third play dealing with AIDS, *The Destiny of Me*, in which the playwright's alter ego, Ned Weeks, is a patient of Dr. Anthony Della Vida at a federal medical research facility that has just become the target of the AIDS-activist organization that Ned has helped found. Ned and Tony greet each other as Ned is admitted:

TONY: Hello, you monster!

NED: I never understand why you talk to me . . .

TONY: I'm very fond of you.

NED: . . . after all I say about you.

and they discuss the experimental treatment:

TONY: Nothing works for everybody.

NED: Nobody believes you.

TONY: Then why are you here?

NED: I'm more desperate. And you sold me a bill of goods.

TONY: You begged me [sic] you were ready to try anything. (Act I)

After he is admitted to the research hospital and is alone, Ned laments: "When we were on the outside, fighting to get in, it was easier to call everyone names. But they were smart. They invited us inside. And we saw they looked human. And that makes hate harder" (Act 1). As Kramer would later remark in an interview with *Diseased Pariah News*, "I think one of the biggest mistakes AIDS activists made was going inside and becoming a part of the system . . . because it's harder to be harsh on people when you actually sit there and work with them all the time on a personal level." This "kinder, gentler" Ned Weeks, however, did not prevent Kramer from characterizing Fauci as a "complete failure" and "the great pretender" in two essays in the nationally circulated lesbian and gay magazine, *The Advocate* in late 1993, a year after *The Destiny of Me* opened in New York's Greenwich Village. Once again, language failed Kramer when he could not transform the rhetoric he used to get people's attention into another set of rhetorical tools that would facilitate his work among AIDS policy leaders and bureaucrats.[29]

Kramer and his critics have tended to psychologize this failure. While I would not dismiss outright a psychoanalytic critique, the problem can also be understood as a social semiotic phenomenon. Kramer had acquired the confrontational "habitus," in Bourdieu's terminology, that is to say "socially constructed dispositions . . . which imply a certain propensity to speak and to say determinate things (the expressive interest) and a certain capacity to speak, which involves both the linguistic capacity to generate an infinite number of grammatically correct discourses, and the social capacity to use this competence adequately in a determinate situation." This habitus for Bourdieu is associated with what he calls a "bodily hexis," that is the very way we physically present ourselves in different situations, a mode of presentation that, like the linguistic habitus, is socially constructed and adaptable and that also, like linguistic discourse, can be "read."[30] Anyone who has seen Kramer speak, yell, scowl, whine, and cringe knows these ways of (re)presenting his body; they are to a great degree learned and arise from his own social (family, ethnic, class) circumstances: an insider outsider. This position becomes apparent not only from Kramer's journalistic frankness about his life, but was dramatically realized in his most recent and revealing play, *The Destiny of Me*.

If that's the way he treats his friends, what about his enemies? In his 1985 play, *The Normal Heart*, Kramer took aim at numerous targets: federal, state, and city leadership; the medical establishment; the media. With its stage set a billboard for AIDS statistics and other pertinent facts, the play was virtually a *pièce à clef*.[31] In the play's first scene, Kramer's alter ego, Ned Weeks, a gay journalist, has gone to see physician Dr. Emma Brookner because of his concerns about "gay cancer." Brookner identifies the culprits:

> EMMA: This hospital sent its report of our first cases to the medical journals over a year ago. *The New England Journal of Medicine* has finally published it, and last week, which brought you running, the *Times* ran something on some inside page. Very inside: page twenty. If you remember, Legionnaire's Disease, toxic shock, they both hit the front page of the *Times* the minute they happened. And stayed there until somebody did something. The front page of the *Times* has a way of inspiring action. . . . You have a Commissioner of Health who got burned with the Swine Flu epidemic, declaring an emergency when there wasn't one. The government appropriated $150 million for that mistake. You have a Mayor who's a bachelor and I assume afraid of being perceived as too friendly to anyone gay. And who is also out to protect a billion-dollar-a-year tourist industry. He's not about to tell the world there's an epidemic menacing his city. And don't ask me about the President. Is the Mayor gay?
>
> NED: If he is, like J. Edgar Hoover, who would want him?

Later in the play Ned summarizes "his" recent article in the *New York Native* (a paraphrase of one of Kramer's essays):

> NED: I said we're all cowards! I said rich gays will give thousands to straight charities before they'll give us a dime. I said it is appalling that some twenty million men and women don't have one single lobbyist in

Washington. How do we expect to achieve anything, ever, at all, by immaculate conception? I said the gay leaders who created this sexual-liberation philosophy in the first place have been the death of us. (II, 9)

When Emma requests federal funding to support her work with over 2,000 cases of AIDS, the reviewing physician turns down her request because her research has been "imprecise and unfocused":

EMMA: . . . What am I arguing with you for? You don't know enough medicine to treat a mouse. You don't know enough science to study boiled water. How dare you come and judge me?

EXAMINING DOCTOR: We only serve on this panel at the behest of Dr. Joost.

EMMA: Another idiot. And, by the way, a closeted homosexual who is doing everything in his power to sweep this under the rug, and I vowed I'd never say that in public. How does it always happen that all the idiots are always on your team? You guys have all the money, call the shots, shut everybody out, and then operate behind closed doors. . . . Your National Institutes of Health received my first request for research money two years ago. It took you one year just to print up application forms. It's taken you two and a half years from my first reported case just to show up here to take a look. The paltry amount of money you are making us beg for—from the four billion dollars you are given each and every year—won't come to anyone until only God knows when. Any way you add this up, it is an unconscionable delay and has never, never existed in any other health emergency during this entire century. While something is being passed around that causes death. We are enduring an epidemic of death. . . . We could all be dead before you do anything. You want my patients? Take them! TAKE THEM! (*She starts hurling her folders and papers at him, out into space.*) Just do something for them! You're fucking right I'm imprecise and unfocused. And you are all idiots! (II, 12)

In one of the play's later scenes, Kramer re-presented his own ejection from Gay Men's Health Crisis (GMHC), the AIDS service organization he helped found, when Ned receives a letter from the board of directors of the organization he has started:

"You are on a colossal ego trip we must curtail. To manipulate fear, as you have done repeatedly in your 'merchandising' of this epidemic, is to us a gesture of barbarism. To exploit the deaths of gay men, as you have done in publications all over America, is to us an act of inexcusable vandalism. And to attempt to justify your bursts of outrageous temper as 'part of what it means to be Jewish" is past our comprehending. And, after years of liberation, you have helped make sex dirty again for us—terrible and forbidden. (II, 13)

In an introduction to his second play, *Just Say No: A Play About a Farce*, Kramer offered this explanation for the level of his invective in *The Normal Heart*: "Why was I going after the *New York Times*? Because, along with Koch and Reagan, they shared an ignoble disdain for AIDS. . . . And [*The Normal Heart*'s producer] Joe Papp and Joe Papp's lawyers joined with me in offering on a stage the dramatic argument: AIDS was originally allowed to grow and grow and grow because the Mayor of New York is a closeted homosexual so terrified of being uncovered that he would rather allow an epidemic" (xxi, xxii).

In *Just Say No*, Kramer employed satire and ridicule over invective. The action revolves around a conspiracy between the Mrs. Potentate (the wife of a president, referred to only as "Daddy") and her "hag fag" Foppy Schwartz. Foppy is a comic version of Roy Cohn, the homosexual who has sold his birthright for a mess of Republican pottage. And the first scene of the play, in which Foppy is furiously answering several phones at once in an effort to "dish" the latest "dirt" would be echoed a few years later in Tony Kushner's first-act scene introducing the Cohn character in *Angels in America: Millennium Approaches*. The moral voice of the play is Foppy's black housekeeper who addresses the audience in a prologue:

> Listen my children, and you shall hear
> How we came to be screwed so drear
> By Mommy and Daddy, who make all the rules,
> And then live by other ones—making us fools.
> Yet some of us have survived the worst.
> We got out alive, although we are cursed
> For letting them flimflam us yet once again,
> And again and again and again and again.
> Someday we'll learn, that's this woman's plea.
> So I tell you this story to help us all see
> How we tried to fight, though given the shaft,
> By their mob of the powerful, brutal, and daft.
> A trivial comedy, Oscar once said,
> But for serious people, before we are dead. [32]

Foppy is a procurer for the closeted Mayor of "Big Appleburg" ("The Mayor still has difficulty sustaining anything . . . permanent? He is too old to be so choosy. And ugly. He's much too ugly. And mean. He's dreadfully mean" [Act I]) the northeast's largest city, who visits Foppy's home for an assignation. In the play's second act, Eustacia taunts the Mayor:

EUSTACIA: . . . How come you starve so many homeless?

MAYOR: They're not hungry. They're demented. Look, if you feel guilty, see a priest . . .

EUSTACIA: . . . How come so many people on your payroll taking kick-backs? Crime and murder and manslaughter at new historic heights?

MAYOR: You're very nosy. My people love me. They stand in line to picket me. I thought down South you people knew your place.

EUSTACIA: . . . My people hate you. My people are going to kill you. There are more of my people than you think. You better not run for another term.

MAYOR: Voodoo politics. . . . Your Jesse keeps stirring up the schvartzahs, I got enough bigoted whites to get me reelected. I got a black police chief, they can't accuse me of racism.

With dialogue like this, who needs comedy? *Just Say No* was Kramer's least well received play, and perhaps for that reason was his favorite; he attributed its box-office failure to a "hateful" *New York Times* review.[33]

Kramer's purpose in writing *Just Say No* was "to find yet another way to expose our two most active murderers, Reagan and Koch, and hope that people would hear me." Koch had been Kramer's and other activist's target for many years. By the end of the decade, Kramer would write: "I hate and loathe Ed Koch with every fiber of my being and every ounce of energy I have. And so should every single gay man and lesbian in New York City. And so should every person touched by AIDS in New York City—gay, straight, white, black, hispanic, man, woman, child." When Koch ran for a fourth term, he lost to David Dinkins, "a mayor as weak as Koch was obnoxious." Even the 1992 election of a publicly gay-friendly Democrat to the White House did not appease Kramer for long; three months after Bill Clinton's inauguration, at a dinner honoring Donna Shalala, secretary of the Department of Health and Human Services, he circulated a flyer with the headline: "Donna Do-Nothing Works for Bill the Welsher," which argued that Clinton had not fulfilled his promise to appoint an "AIDS czar."[34]

Kramer acknowledged the pariah status of gays and lesbians in America, to which he attributed the lack of progress in handling the AIDS epidemic. In a speech at a symposium on the Constitution, Kramer took the opportunity to assert that "the AIDS pandemic is the fault of the white, middle-class, male majority. AIDS is here because the straight world would not grant equal rights to gay people. If we had been allowed to get married, to have legal rights, there would be no AIDS cannonballing through America." And once again he named names: "that horrible monster, Robert Bork, or that equally horrible monster, the dogma of the Catholic Church . . . the Right Wing, the Moral Majority, fundamentalists, Mormons, Southern Baptists, born-agains, Orthodox Jews, Hasidic Jews, La Rouchies, Jesse Helms, Representative Dannemeyer, Governor Deukmejian, Phyllis Schlafly, Jerry Falwell, enemies all." His argument was that since a heterosexual dominant culture had forbidden gay and lesbian people from entering legal marriages, gays and lesbians became sexual dissidents who embraced the function of erotic pariahs.[35]

In that regard, Kramer represented himself both as a middle-class exemplar and as a pariah, or as I formulated it above, an insider outsider. His writing often seems self-congratulatory and self-promoting, frequently noting his Yale alma mater, his film-world successes, his writing achievements, his brother the lawyer, and his search for a committed relationship. On the one hand, these might be ethical appeals, in terms of Classical rhetoric, establishing his credibility to a largely middle-class, educated audience of power brokers in business, law, government, and medicine. On the other, they signify Kramer's own multiple, competing subject positions and the ambiguities and contradictions inherent in AIDS politics and gay identity politics. He further (dis)placed himself in a marginal position, first by acknowledging that he is gay, second by acknowledging that he is HIV positive, and third by employing confrontational language that situated himself and his subjects or his audiences in opposition to each other. This is not simply a matter of Kramer's wanting it both ways or of being mercurial. Rather, like any HIV infected gay man, Kramer was already socially (and therefore discursively) constructed as deviant, and in America, deviance (especially sexual deviance, which is also always to say "medical") is configured as dangerous to health. Likewise, the tradition of the jeremiad virtually compelled him to position himself in opposition; regardless of what legislators, bureau-crats, or medical researchers contribute, it is never enough for the jeremiadic preacher.

APOCALYPTIC CRISIS

Because a constellation of medical disorders appeared to coalesce around gay men residing in the West Village and Chelsea, Kramer's first audience was other gay men. Eventually as awareness grew of the extent of the "Gay Men's Health Crisis," activists would need to reach larger and less accessible audiences, including elected officials, bureaucrats, and scien-tists.[36] And that task would eventually require access to and coverage by a variety of mass media; in order to compete for audiences' attention and to motivate their action, Kramer would produce large, loud, and repeated signifiers of apocalyptic crisis.

Kramer tapped into a crisis discourse already existing for his audi-ence. The Anita Bryant "Save Our Children" campaign in the late 1970s had elicited a sense of urgency from many gay and lesbian activists around the country. The 1980 presidential election of Ronald Reagan came about in part because of the support of a conservative religious coalition calling itself "The Moral Majority," headed by Christian fundamentalist pastor Jerry Falwell, which advanced an antigay social agenda. As Rodger Streitmatter documents, antigay campaigns had become material of na-tional news reporting, including reports of legislative initiatives to insti-tute the death penalty for homosexual acts and a censoring of the gay press.[37] In December 1980, the *New York Native*, initially printed in tabloid format, began publication with front-page headlines equal to the city's tabloid rhetoric: "The West Street Massacre," which posed the question, "Has the Moral Majority sent its first commando into the gay community?" A lone gunman had entered the Ramrod, New York's "butchest" gay men's bar, shooting and killing or wounding many of the customers. An advertisement early in the decade for the newly-formed National Gay Task Force announced: "They're out to kill! If you are gay or lesbian, you are the target for right wing political opportunists and religious fanatics."[38]

If Kramer's entry into AIDS activism, one might almost say his "invention" of AIDS activism, was marked by restraint—the notice in the August 24, 1981 issue of the *New York Native* began, "It's difficult to write this without sounding alarmist or too emotional or just plain scared" (and Robert Chesley's characterization of it as "alarmist" not withstanding), Kramer's rhetoric would become gradually more urgent during the next two years. In the fall of 1982, for example, in a column for the second newsletter of GMHC, Kramer would characterize the medical situation in these terms: "[I]t is hard to imagine a worse emergency, or an enemy to match the stealth and horror of this insidious epidemic, an unknown disease that hides itself." Less than a year later in March 1983, Kramer would issue his most famous jeremiad, "1,112 and Counting," which warned: "Our continued existence as gay men upon the face of this earth is at stake. Unless we fight for our lives, we shall die. In all the history of homosexuality we have never before been so close to death and extinction." Kramer produced his most striking apocalyptic sign, genocide, by overlaying an American history of heterosexist violence with this century's Nazi "Final Solution" that had resulted in the Holocaust.[39]

Gay people's fears of a right-wing purge or genocide of homosexuals predated the AIDS crisis. First, it has historical analogues in medieval, Renaissance, and early modern Europe where sodomy convictions were punishable by death. In the twentieth century, Nazis had incarcerated homosexuals in the death camps. Even more recently, John Francis Hunter's 1971 *The Gay Insider: A Hunter's Guide to New York and a Thesaurus of Phallic Lore*, says of the perennial Greenwich Village neighborhood bar, Julius: "When every other gay bar goes under, which won't happen, I keep *saying*, unless the Fascists take over or the straight puritanical revolutionaries succeed (at which point we might as well all haul ass to Canada, as there would be gay genocide one way or the other), Julius will probably hang on." A novel published a decade later by Alabama Birdstone, *Queer Free*, is an account of gradual repression and finally internment of homosexuals in the United States. Later in the decade novelist Tim Barrus would make the connection between AIDS and government repression with his fiction sequence, *Genocide: The Anthology*.[40]

From the beginning, Kramer linked urgency with action. As the scope of the epidemic became more obvious to Kramer and others, the need for concerted action on the part of all gay men became clear. "I am sick of closeted gays," Kramer announced,

> It's 1983 already, guys, when are you going to come out? By 1984 you could be dead. Every gay man who is unable to come forward now and fight to save his own life is truly helping to kill the rest of us. There

is only one thing that's going to save some of us, and this is *numbers* and pressure and our being perceived as united and a threat. As more and more of my friends die, I have less and less sympathy for men who are afraid their mommies will find out or afraid their bosses will find out or afraid their fellow doctors or professional associates will find out. Unless we can generate, visibly, numbers, masses, we are going to die.

Even two years into the official epidemic, many New York gay men resisted Kramer's urgency; as he noted: "I am sick of everyone in this community who tells me to stop creating a panic. How many of us have to die before *you* get scared off your ass and into action?" And Kramer made explicit the homology he saw between the Holocaust and AIDS:

I am sick of "men" who say, 'We've got to keep quiet or *they* will do such and such." *They* usually means the straight majority, the "Moral" Majority, or similarly perceived representatives of *them*. Okay, you "men"—be my guests: You can march off now to the gas chambers; just get right in line.[41]

Not surprisingly, responses at the time to this essay were mixed. Although some letters to the editor acknowledged his effectiveness in getting them to do something—write a check to GMHC or examine their own sexual behavior—others condemned his crisis rhetoric. A lengthy response by Ralph Sepulveda, Jr., for example, asserted that, "The philosophy behind Mr. Kramer's piece seems to be that in times like these, when drastic actions must be taken, drastic words must also be spoken, and so he goes all out. But surely he goes too far when he turns his rhetorical overkill against us, his gay readers, and begins assailing us as though *we* (!) were the enemy. . . . [I]n order to spur people to action, he finds it necessary to rush out and spread guilt and fear and panic over the land." Jim Levin characterized Kramer as an "*arriviste* to the gay community without a sense of history" and his essay as "most inaccurate and most harmful." Christopher Lynn saw Kramer's growing visibility and stridency as self-serving, accusing him of trying first to merchandise his novel *Faggots* and now to merchandise AIDS. But perhaps the most carefully antiapocalyptic critique of Kramer's language in this essay came in a letter from Jurg Mahner:

We are not under the threat of being wiped out as a community. The Holocaust atmosphere Larry is creating in his article I consider as being

as dangerous to ourselves as when we created the Mineshaft and the
Lofts [two men's bars] to live there our fantasies instead of trying to
come to grip with them by less dangerous means. We have a health-
problem on an impressive scale. But it was not designed by evil forces
to destroy us and nobody talks about herding us into camps or to put
triangles on our bomber-jackets apart from those we put there volun-
tarily. To imply that the straight world is ready, or will soon be ready
to do anything of that sort is an insult to all of those straight men who
are on our side and do support us although they have difficulties to
swallow some of our excesses like fucking in public on summer Sun-
days on the sidewalks of West Highway. *We are not* under the threat of
extinction and to say so I regard as another expression of the very
feeling of being victims Larry Kramer tries to tell us to get rid of.

Lending credibility to Mahner's position was the fact that he had recently
been hospitalized for an AIDS-related illness and reported favorably on
his medical treatment, in addition to the fact that as a self-described
"foreigner" he stood at a remove from the American tradition of apocalyptic crisis.[42]

In the summer of 1983, Kramer vacationed in Europe and visited
Dachau, where, he would say later, "the thoughts began to coalesce into
what would shortly become my play *The Normal Heart.*" When the
play opened in the spring of 1985, the simple stage set served as billboards for important data related to the AIDS epidemic. One wall,
however, presented a lengthy quotation from *American Jewry During the
Holocaust*, a report published in 1984 by the American Jewish Commission on the Holocaust:

> There were two alternative strategies a Jewish organization could adopt
> to get the American government to initiate action on behalf of the
> imperiled Jews of Europe. It could cooperate with the government
> officials, quietly trying to convince them that rescue of Jews should be
> one of the objectives of the war, or it could try to pressure the govern-
> ment into initiating rescue by using embarrassing public attention and
> rallying public opinion to that end. The American Jewish Committee
> chose the former strategy and clung to it tenaciously. . . . They were
> still trying to persuade the same officials when the war ended.[43]

In the play, Kramer's alter ego, Ned Weeks, wonders aloud at how the
U.S. government maintained silence concerning the fate of European
Jews from 1933 until the 1944 publication of Treasury Secretary

Morgenthau's report to President Roosevelt, *Acquiescence of This Government in the Murder of the Jews* (I.iv). This knowledge produces a paranoia leading one of the play's characters, Mickey, to observe:

> I used to love my country. The *Native* received an anonymous letter describing top-secret Defense Department experiments at Fort Detrick, Maryland, that have produced a virus that can destroy the immune system. Its code name is Firm Hand. They started testing in 1978—on a group of gays. I never used to believe shit like this before. They are going to persecute us! Cancel our health insurance. Test our blood to see if we're pure. Lock us up. Stone us in the streets. (II xi)

As outrageous as this delusion appears, it is fairly tame compared to some that circulated at the time when the etiology of AIDS was still uncertain.[44] Kramer also captures some of the medical urgency at the time in the character of Dr. Emma Brookner, a physician disabled by polio who requires a wheelchair. While she does not explicitly employ the trope of AIDS as genocide, Emma does project an AIDS cataclysm: "I am seeing more cases each week than the week before. I figure that by the end of the year the number will be doubling every six months. That's something over a thousand cases by next June. Half of them will be dead. Your two friends I've just diagnosed? One of them will be dead. Maybe both of them" (I I).

With respect to capturing and keeping an audience's attention, once you've proclaimed viral genocide, where do you go from there? If Kramer's jeremiad could hardly have become more alarmist from the mid 1980s, its alarmism could at least be reproduced repeatedly and joined with a demonization of the "enemy." Kramer continued with the AIDS body count in such articles as "2,339 and Counting," published in 1983 in the *Village Voice*, a progressive paper that focuses on downtown and alternative culture, and "100,000 and Counting," published later in 1989 in the short-lived but significant gay weekly, *Outweek*. Concluding this last essay, Kramer wrote,

> Oh, I have said all of this so many times and for so long. But I have no choice but to say all of it again. So, for those of you who have been reading my words over these past long years, now that we have reached that awful and awe-ful number of 100,000, there is nothing new I can bring to solemnize its arrival. I am still the one-note wailer. I'm grateful I'm still able to be here screaming, and I'm grateful I'm joined by many

more screamers than were around when I started my caterwauling another lifetime ago. But I sure wish, as I've prayed from the beginning, *everybody* else was screaming too. We're heading for the last roundup, boys and girls. How many men and women are willing to stand up and be counted, at last?

In a later reflection on his 1988 "Open Letter Dr. Anthony Fauci," Kramer admitted self-reflexively, "The level of rhetoric gets higher, the pitch more shrill," as though he himself recognized the hyperbole, but was unable to adapt that discourse to different situations.[45]

On several occasions Kramer expressed a desire for violent action, though admitting that he would not be its agent. In an essay for *Outweek* magazine in March 1990, Kramer called for "a MASSIVE DISRUPTION of the Sixth International AIDS Conference . . . in San Francisco." Turning up the volume, Kramer asserted, "WE HAVE BEEN LINED UP IN FRONT OF A FIRING SQUAD, AND IT IS CALLED AIDS. WE MUST RIOT! I AM CALLING FOR A FUCKING RIOT!" Later reflecting on this manifesto, Kramer would admit, "I hadn't given much thought to just what I meant by 'riot.' . . . I didn't mean violence, though I can see where it's possible to read into my text that, if you are prone to it, by all means . . ."[46] In a 1994 interview with *Diseased Pariah News*, Kramer would admit:

> It comes down to the fact that we are being murdered, and we are being murdered intentionally, and in my book that equals genocide. So one man's line is not another man's in terms of how you respond to all of that. I wish to hell there were some people out there courageous and crazy enough to go out there and throw bombs or burn buildings, or put a mark on Jesse Helms, or whatever. But for whatever reason we don't represent a population that's in any way capable of doing that. . . . So how do you draw a line? I don't know. I am not capable myself of taking a gun and shooting somebody, not even as an undercover vigilante—but I wish to fuck I was capable of it. And I keep saying I hope there's somebody out there who is.[47]

Kramer was employing a militant discourse that became common among many AIDS and queer activists in the early 1990s, which I will discuss in the next chapter. However, having begun at a high pitch in the early 1980s, he found it increasingly difficult to make credible assertions about the health crisis. In response to the *Diseased Pariah News* interview, socialist Scott Tucker maintained that "Kramer's assimilationist cultural politics are only the reverse image of his apocalyptic anarchism" and he asked, "Is Kramer such a drama queen that he does not understand the risk of his own performances?"[48] In the American "marketplace of ideas" (a "liberal" phrase that betrays our consumerist structures while it belies the incommensurability of ideas with material production) such extreme language is usually either contained (and thus marginalized) or co-opted. I think a bit of both happened to Kramer, who eventually became the "talking head" or media personality that producers call when they want to "balance" a panel of "policy wonks," knowing that he will say something incendiary, but won't bring a gun and start shooting in the studio. In some ways, the only thing worse in America than being ignored is getting in a television news producer's Rolodex. Kramer's discourse, both in its oppositional and crisis tropes, has become a stereotype; although he continued to appear in a variety of news media during the 1990s, it was as a caricature of himself. As a result, his words were no longer as effective as they once were.

The 1989 publication of *Reports from the Holocaust*, and an expanded edition in 1994, permitted Kramer to compose longer, more reflective and less tactical essays that frequently detailed the trope of genocide. These essays were informed in part by the writing of philosophers and scholars like Hannah Arendt, Primo Levi, John Boswell, Zygmunt Bauman, and Ernest Becker.[49] In these essays Kramer worked out more carefully his understanding of AIDS and genocide. In the first edition's "Report from the Holocaust" Kramer narrated his own life in the AIDS epidemic and the questions about which he had come to some conclusions, including, "Why has the straight world, by and large, been unable to face or cope with the realities of what is happening to us—to such a degree that I now believe some form of intentional genocide is going on?" In asserting a gay Holocaust, however, Kramer waffled with the same ambivalence he felt for Anthony Fauci. On the one hand, he believed that "genocide is occurring: that we are witnessing—or *not* witnessing—the systematic, planned annihilation of some by others with the avowed purpose of eradicating an undesirable portion of the population"; on the other hand, "a holocaust does not require *deliberate* intentionality on the part of one or several or many or a bureaucracy to be effective. Holocausts can occur, and probably most often do occur, because of *inaction*. This inaction can be unintentional or deliberate." In an essay prepared for the 1994 revised edition of this collection, Kramer would still admit,

Yes, I speak in hyperbole, and yes, I speak the truth. Yes, there's been progress, and no, there's been no progress. Yes, people are living longer because some doctors know how to keep us alive longer . . . and patients have a better understanding of how to take care of themselves. . . . No, there still remain so many unanswered questions on the pathogenesis of AIDS . . .

And he would conclude: "Official genocide is going on."[50]

Kramer was more and more frequently invited to speak on campuses and at other gatherings where he took advantage of the opportunity to speak in blunt terms to those assembled, calling for grassroots activism that led to the formation of ACT UP, speaking at annual Gay Pride gatherings, even speaking at memorial services. Kramer also moved toward a militant discourse, calling for an AIDS "Manhattan Project," oddly reconfiguring the identity of the military-scientific project that ushered in the apocalyptic nuclear age, and calling for an "AIDS High Command."[51] At an event marking the tenth anniversary of GMHC held in the Episcopal Cathedral of St. John the Divine, Kramer would claim, "here I am telling you that everything we have done and we are doing is useless and that we have no choice but to start all over again in our fight." Receiving an award from Body Positive as "Person of the Year" in 1990, Kramer announced he was leaving AIDS and gay activism, since "We have lost the war against AIDS . . . and in our utter despair, we make each other the enemy." Even at the memorial service for activist and film historian Vito Russo, Kramer took the occasion to implicate everyone present: "We killed Vito. . . . Everyone in this room killed him. . . . Vito was killed by 25 million gay men and lesbians who for ten long years of this plague have refused to get our act together." While early in the epidemic he had trusted that confrontation with the grim statistics of AIDS would move people from their apathy and passivity, by 1993 he was telling students at Yale University (his alma mater) and on other campuses that even this tactic had failed to be effective:

I only say one thing in my speeches now. I say it over and over and over wherever I can and to whomever will listen or interview me or put my loud unpleasant presence on TV. . . . This is what I say. AIDS is intentional genocide. It is intentional. It is intentional. It is intentional genocide and I know with all my heart and soul that it is intentional and I am not going to spend any more time giving you chapter and verse on the whys and wherefores. Read my book . . . AIDS

is intentional genocide. AIDS is intentional genocide. AIDS is intentional genocide. AIDS is intentional genocide. AIDS is intentional
genocide. AIDS is intentional genocide. . . . Genocide is a crime an
entire society commits. Genocide is a crime an entire society commits. Genocide is a crime an entire society commits. Genocide is a
crime an entire society commits.[52]

As though surrendering the possibility of rationally proving genocide,
Kramer resorted to an obsessive repetition of the simplest reduction of
his message, an oratorical metonymy of ACT UP demonstration graphics
asserting Silence = Death or wheat-pasted advertising bills on walls
throughout the city endlessly repeated, in other words, the "sound bite"
as the verbal equivalent of the image in the world of signs. Getting
someone in New York City to notice a message and messenger requires
attention to size and repetition: signifiers must be "big" or attention
getting and they must be endlessly reproduced. The result is a kind of
saturation, and admittedly one that reaches a point of diminishing return, where the audience simply becomes over-familiarized with the
message and then stops noticing it. I suspect that this was the case with
Kramer who, although he continued to appear on television talk shows
and on conference panels as well as in the pages of the *Times*, the *Washington Post*, and other high profile periodicals, did not receive the same
attentive listening, though it was nonetheless a respectful listening. When
I met him in New York in February of 1996, Kramer seemed avuncular
to the students gathered at a City University of New York symposium.
However, AIDS has long been colonized under the aegis of public policy,
a discursive zone that Kramer admitted he had neither the interest nor
the background for, which he has ably demonstrated.

APOCALYPTIC AFFIRMATION

Although his most striking language has concerned a binary demonization
of "enemies" and evocation of apocalyptic crisis, Kramer's activism has
fairly consistently returned to several affirmations: the dignity of gay
people, the value of monogamous partnerships, the need for gay community, and the possibility of reform and renewal. All of these are fairly
mainstream middle class American values; Kramer has never claimed to
be a sexual or social radical. Because of his predictable excoriation of

groups and individuals, these affirmations are generally all the more re-markable. For example, the last scene of *The Normal Heart* is a marriage of Felix and Ned witnessed by Dr. Brookner before Felix dies. The au-dience witnesses the double layering of Western dramatic conventions: the marriage scene of comedy and the death-bed scene of melodrama. This layering is not simply an interesting formal device, since it signified Kramer's ambiguous subjectivity. The marriage scene represents bour-geois inclusion; the death-bed scene, the sign of the outcast who must be sacrificed. Both scenes, however, tend to assume a bourgeois audience. Similarly, at the end of *The Destiny of Me*, a substantially wiser play though no less angry, Ned affirms life and asserts the redemptive power of love, reconciling his past (the memory of his childhood self, Alexander) with his present and future:

ALEXANDER: . . . What's going to happen to me?

NED: You're going to go to eleven shrinks. You won't fall in love for forty years. And when a nice man finally comes along and tries to teach you to love him and love yourself, he dies from a plague. Which is waiting to kill you, too.

ALEXANDER: I'm sorry I asked. Do I learn anything?

NED: Does it make any sense, a life? (*Singing.*) "Only make believe I love you . . ."

ALEXANDER: (*Singing.*) "Only make believe that you love me . . ."

NED: When Felix was offered the morphine drip for the first time in the hospital, I asked him, "Do you want it now or later?" Felix somehow found the strength to answer back, "I want to stay a little longer."

NED and ALEXANDER: "Might as well make believe I love you . . ."

NED: "For to tell the truth . . ."

NED and ALEXANDER: "I do."

NED: I want to stay a little longer. (Act III)

This "I do" echoes the exchange of vows at the end of the earlier play and signifies the possibility of "marrying" or unifying fragmented subject positions as well as a utopian closure of desire, dramatic strategies that would not be unfamiliar to most audience members. In that respect, the play's ending engages a whole repertoire of our stereotypical reactions to romantic comedy. In a 1994 interview, Kramer asserted:

> I think everyone's capable of great and wonderful love, and I think everybody wants that. . . . I just think it's sad—and this is a moral thing, I'm not going to deny that I'm moral about it—I think it's sad that so much of the energy of this wonderful community had to go to sex, to the exclusion of everything else, to the exclusion of building a political movement, fighting for rights for gay men and lesbians, getting and maintaining power in the political process. Would that the gay political movement had available to it the brains and the caliber of professional people fighting to establish this movement [as those] who would go off to the baths. [53]

Both Ian Young and Douglas Sadownick later came to argue a similar point. In *The Stonewall Experiment: A Gay Psychohistory* Young contends that the post-Stonewall gay ghetto and its erotic excesses were little more than gay men's adoption of one of the dominant culture's more pernicious myths linking homosexuality with death. While less critical of Dionysian eroticism, Sadownick's *Sex between Men: An Intimate History of the Sex Lives of Gay Men Postwar to Present* argues from a post-Jungian perspective that gay men often literalize and externalize in the men they desire what they would be better off seeking within themselves.[54] The publication of both of these books suggests a shift in AIDS discourse (though it was always present) toward the local and personal, away from the political. American politics entails a host of compromises: strange bedfellows and Faustian bargains that go against the grain of American idealism. We would rather flee by going West; or when that option is no longer open to us, by turning inward. By the mid-1990s many activists had grown tired of shouting, became policy bureaucrats, or died. Kramer's ambivalence about his eventual inclusion in AIDS policy making is not simply a tactical reservation. The jeremiad underwrites a Romantic idealism that cannot remain true to itself within the realm of the political with its compromises and cooptations. Discursively, when Kramer lost his innocence and fell into politics, he had the jeremiad at his disposal as ritual atonement. However, while no social movement and its discourse can remain "pure" or persist long in rage, Kramer's moral vision remained fairly consistent, even when his demonization and evocation of crisis became more pitched.

KRAMER'S RECEPTION

Larry Kramer's jeremiads have reached a variety of audiences, including participants in Gay Pride parades, readers of lesbian and gay periodicals, theater audiences, as well as the readers of the *Times* and the *Wall Street Journal.* Their responses, as characterized by the narrative of his entry into activism that I have provided, have been predictably varied.

The critical reception of his plays has been frequently split, as Joel Shatzky demonstrates with regard to *The Normal Heart.* New York critics' reactions to Kramer's first AIDS-issue play "indicate that unlike many plays that are judged on the basis of aesthetic qualities in terms of script, production, and performance, . . . *The Normal Heart* had created an audience that attended as much to the political and social content . . ." as to its dramatic form. While characterizing *The Normal Heart* as "more of a tract than a play," New York critic Clive Barnes admitted,

> Yet even if it is primarily an essay in pamphleteering, a nobly partisan polemic, that does not mean that what Kramer is saying is not worth saying. And how many people of the thousands who will see the play, and be stirred by its sheer intensity and passionate concern, would ever have read the tract? Here . . . the theater is not just standing there. It is doing something. It is shouting. And it behooves us to listen.

Concerning the form of the play, D. S. Lawson asserted that "Kramer wisely jettisons conventional realism; since he wishes to indict the society in which he places his characters, he does not wish to support that society by using a set of dramatic conventions that have long served that very society's interests." In an analysis that compares Andrew Holleran's pre-AIDS novel about Fire Island, *Dancer from the Dance,* with Randy Shilts's novelistic AIDS history, *And the Band Played On,* and Kramer's play, James Miller constructs "a fundamentalist canon of plague scriptures for which there is not precedent in secular literature: a Gay Old Testament," which Miller characterizes as "Holleran's Fall myth . . . Shilts's Chronicles . . . Kramer's Lamentations." Thus, I suppose for some critics, the sins of the novel were visited upon the plays. In the introduction to an anthology of

AIDS plays edited by M. Elizabeth Osborn (which does not include *The Normal Heart* because Kramer withheld it), Michael Feingold suggested that this play "just by virtue of its aggressive position-taking on the subject, . . . [has] already had many useful effects, among them the gift of provoking censorship battles which have revealed—as if we didn't already know—that the American public, in 1990, remains as confused and un-informed about the nature of art as about that of AIDS" In his *Village Voice* review of Kramer's later play, *The Destiny of Me*, Feingold added concerning the first: "[I]t did provoke controversy, a public airing of gay anger and frustration at everyone's failure to do more, an increased determination to fight. Its productions since have probably done a good deal to raise the level of public awareness about the plague." Kramer has been a polemical writer ever since *Faggots*. As a result, instead of being compelled to retain some kind of formalist "purity" in *The Normal Heart* in order to produce a sentimentally lyrical play, Kramer "fell into" politics dramatically. In this regard, Kramer's play distinguished itself from William Hoffman's more elegiac *As Is*. In some respects it was precisely because of his willingness to be boldly political that we listened to him in the mid-1980s and that we tended to ignore him by the mid-1990s.[55]

Critical reception was similarly split over *The Destiny of Me*, includ-ing imperious New York critics at both ends, from Clive Barnes's dis-missal ("a self-indulgent play") to John Simon's rave ("may be the most comprehending, and is certainly the most comprehensive, AIDS play so far"). While critics generally agreed that all three of Kramer's plays were seriously flawed—in terms of structure, language, and diction—most also concurred that their impact had been immense in bringing AIDS to public awareness.[56]

The Normal Heart and *The Destiny of Me* are so transparently auto-biographical that even Larry Kramer's published essays and speeches come out of the mouths of his characters. In several instances, when characters of the plays quote the character "Ned Weeks" they are quoting Kramer's previously published essays. The world of journalistic discourse thus in-sinuated itself into the venue of dramatic discourse. Audience members for these *pièces à clef* responded simultaneously to the virtual Ned Weeks and the actual Larry Kramer. As a result, as several critics noted, the plays followed a political aesthetic. As I suggested earlier the personal and the personality are the political. It is thus difficult, if not impossible, to separate one's reactions to the plays from one's reactions to Kramer. With the distinction between the message and the messenger all but evaporated, the reception of Kramer and Kramer's language is easily over-personalized. The ideological lines had already been drawn in hostility to Kramer's novel, *Faggots*, when his first AIDS writing appeared in 1981. Respondents to the *New York Native* had likewise been willing to canonize or to demonize him for his later letters, articles, or statements reported in the news. In some cases, the criticism has been that Kramer himself was demonizing others or that he was creating a self-serving crisis. Over two decades into the epidemic, we now see that the crisis was real, but also that the crisis is more complex than Kramer's binary constructions could adequately represent.

In a study of GMHC and the politics of volunteerism, Philip Kayal criticized Kramer for failing to see the political dimensions of GMHC's services and volunteer involvement and Kramer's willingness to construct enemies:

> Kramer responds to hate with hate and anger. Despite disclaimers, he operates within a traditionally patriarchal political paradigm. [However,] AIDS suggests that radical institutional and personal transformation is necessary so that no group or person will be seen as a dispensable 'other.' . . . In the long run, fighting hate with hate does not resolve anything.[57]

Lee Edelman offered a similar critique from a deconstructive perspective when he interrogated the "simple equations" "Silence = Death" with a bathroom graffito, "Gay Rights = AIDS," and interrogated Kramer's equation of gay political passivity with murder. Edelman suggested that such discourse tends to "reify and absolutize identities" without demanding "critical reading and resistance that call into question *any* equation that represents 'truth' as a literal fact and not as a figural frame." Kramer tended to present sexual identities in essentialist terms, addressing "my people" as though there existed a monolithic gay community, and citing the usual list of history's hundred great homosexuals as though there were among them no nuances of self-understanding, not to mention complex multiple subjectivities constructed by vastly different historical contingencies. Edelman further questioned what difference there was between Pat Buchanan's and Larry Kramer's assertions that gays were killing each other, supporting his contention that discourse on AIDS is always "infected."[58]

Situating Larry Kramer's language in the history of modern queer activism offers another frame of reference. John D'Emilio, for example, acknowledges that the gay liberation movement entailed ambiguities in

which "acts of resistance can unwittingly reproduce, or at least give sus-
tenance to, systems of oppression." Queers (and other marginalized people)
react to legitimate criticism with the same fervor as we react to stigmatizing and demonizing stereotypes. As a result, "the reaction to Larry,
from *Faggots* through AIDS, tells us something important about the
dynamics of gay male sexual culture and sexual politics. To venture into
this territory is like entering a minefield." D'Emilio urges that we view
Kramer as but one activist who happened to be at the right time and
place but who did not exercise the consistent, painstaking work that
results in a social movement. However, he suggests that we also see
Kramer as an unparalleled polemicist whose writing and speeches were
indispensable to advancing AIDS activism. Nonetheless, this work came
at a price for Kramer the Jeremiah:

> For even as his words mobilized, his verbal attacks have also stung and
> have consequently limited the influence he has had on the shape and
> evolution of AIDS policy and on the direction of the gay and lesbian
> movement. As a figure with cultural capital at his disposal, Larry has
> been able to mount a platform from which he can be heard. Yet the
> stance that he has taken—the cultural critic as outsider—necessarily
> creates boundaries around this influence.[59]

Perhaps one of the more sympathetic and careful analyses of Kramer's
discourse came in David Bergman's "Larry Kramer and the Rhetoric of
AIDS," whose goal was to discuss Kramer's plays, essays, letters, and
speeches "not as art but as action. Did he make something happen, or
were his tools unfit for the job? Is he the queen of message queens, or
their ugly stepmother?"[60] Bergman pointed out that Kramer's language
was replete with binary oppositions which Kramer both maintained and
conflated, so that Kramer at Vito Russo's memorial, for example, would
equate less visible or nonactivist gays or lesbians with murderers. The
"vacillation" of maintaining and conflating binarisms, as Sacvan Bercovitch
points out, is a central feature of the jeremiadic ritual with its urgent
idealism and more urgent disappointment.[61] Even Kramer's sympathetic
critics, like Bergman, found it difficult to resist framing their own discourse about him in personal or even psychoanalytic terms, because of
"Kramer's habit of responding to political events as personal affronts,
of transforming impersonal bureaucracies into individual bogeymen, of
subsuming all conflicts into a version of the Freudian family romance
[which] is the source of both the power of his political polemics and of

the problems in them. His broadsides derive much of their creepy insistence from their intimacy." Further, Bergman detected three "family" voices in Kramer's discourse: the enraged child, the guilt-inducing mother, the humiliating father.[62] In some respects, Bergman's psychoanalytic reading reminds me of Richard Hofstadter's characterization of the American paranoid political style. Hofstadter employs the clinical term "paranoid" in a more broadly social sense. While the clinical paranoid "sees the hostile and conspiratorial world in which he feels himself to be living as directed specifically *against him* . . . the spokesman of the paranoid style finds it directed against a nation, a culture, a way of life whose fate affects not himself alone but millions of others." As with Hofstadter's characterization of the paranoid style, Kramer likewise "tend[ed] to be overheated, oversuspicious, overaggressive, grandiose, and apocalyptic in expression."[63] The fact that Hofstadter was able to identify an American cultural pattern suggests that Kramer's activism emerged not simply from a psychological disposition but was enscribed by preexisting paranoid-style discourse. In saying this, however, I do not dismiss Kramer or the seriousness of his concerns, recalling an old joke: Just because you're paranoid doesn't mean everybody *isn't* out to get you. Unconscionable bureaucratic inaction early in the epidemic, an alliance of politicians and government officials with groups who had explicitly targeted gays for social control, and the association of the big-money health care industry interests with conservative causes sometimes makes paranoia seem reasonable.

Therefore, we do not need to resort to psychoanalytic criticism in order to understand Kramer's discourse, for as Sacvan Bercovitch observes:

> American writers have tended to see themselves as outcasts and isolates, prophets crying in the wilderness. So they have been, as a rule: *American* Jeremiahs, simultaneously lamenting a declension and celebrating a national dream. . . . Like the latter-day Puritan Jeremiahs, they could offer *themselves* as the symbol incarnate, and so relocate America— transplant the entire national enterprise, en masse—into the mind and imagination of the exemplary American. . . . To declare oneself the symbol of America is by definition to retain one's allegiance to a middle-class culture. . . . His identification with America as it ought to be impels the writer to withdraw from what it is in America.[64]

Kramer's writing emerged from an existing rhetorical tradition whose binary oppositions and related sense of crisis he employed initially with great effect, understanding himself as "the exemplary American" and managing to maintain his position as an "isolate" when his discursive success had brought him closer to power. Thus following the successful establishment of the first AIDS service organization, Gay Men's Health Crisis, and of a major activist group, ACT UP, Kramer withdrew from each organization and positioned himself as an critical outsider, when they failed, as they had to, to live up to his ideals from them. Furthermore, his insistence on the desirability of homosexual "marriage" marked him as thoroughly middle class, which affiliation also blinded him frequently to the material differences within the "gay community" along lines of gender, race, and class. It also blinded him to the important and effective networks among many of New York's gay men that were produced by nonmonogamous sexual relations. Had they been largely atomized into monogamous "nuclear families" it is uncertain that they would have responded to both the medical and political crises of the 1980s.

Kramer's writing and speaking in the late 1980s and early 1990s was persistently enraged, which "may be the result of his increasing frustration in his failure to find language that is urgent without being oppositional." He announced on several occasions his intention to leave public life or publicly fantasized a violent response to the AIDS crisis, positions for which American jeremiads provide ample precedent.[65] From 1981 until the end of the decade, Kramer's crisis discourse had powerfully effected change on behalf of those affected by AIDS and succeeded in bringing AIDS into public awareness, first among gay men with his journalistic writing and later among ever enlarging circles of people who were awakened by *The Normal Heart*. His persistence in representing AIDS as a crisis eventually contributed to the mobilization of direct action, most visibly in ACT UP. However, both HIV and health care in America have proven to be more complex and recalcitrant than any binary oversimplification can absorb. The tactical effectiveness of Kramer's discourse was thus far less effective at fostering continued action than it was at mobilizing it. Furthermore, by the time of his alienation from ACT UP Kramer had already been implicated in the power structures around AIDS and health care and from which he found it hard to extricate himself discursively. Fond of Dr. Anthony Fauci and accustomed to sharing some measure of power in AIDS-related decision making, he nonetheless continued to identify himself in opposition, vacillating between praise and condemnation in relation to both other AIDS activists and to AIDS bureaucrats. Kramer's combative rhetoric effectively mobilized people threatened with AIDS. However, as the epidemic's politics and economics grew more complex, such martial rhetoric became less useful, creating fictional enemies out of merely overwhelmed bureaucrats.

In the summer of 1995 a new magazine appeared in New York dedicated to the "gay male masses" whom the magazine's editor characterized in the terms of queer anti-assimilationism: "If you are gay, you are not normal. You are not regular, ordinary or everyday. You are weird, you are different, you are threatening and you are definitely queer." Entitled *Lisp*, the magazine claimed as its heritage earlier radical Dada publications and Dada père, Marcel Duchamp, and it declared, "We have no time for 'straight-acting, straight-appearing' cowards, and we really can't be bothered with assimilation. A place has not been set for us at Bruce Bawer's table: we would have the other guests in an instant snit—and we don't like what they are serving for dinner anyway." The transgressive subject position was also apparent in *Lisp*'s back and front covers: on the front, a hand holding a pistol; on the back, a call to arms: "Gay Militias Now Forming . . . because the only arms buildup is not at the gym." In the United States, countercultures often discursively construct themselves as "at war" with the dominant culture (who are usually first constructed as "at war" with the counterculture), in a rhetoric that prepares for the ultimate battle, the American Armageddon. For many in New York City dealing with AIDS was discursively the medical equivalent of war; it is to these martial tropes that I turn in the next chapter.

Chapter Four

AIDS Armageddon

(In memory of Jack,
who always loved a man in uniform)

In its inaugural December 1980 issue, the gay newspaper *New York Native*, which for most of the decade would provide initially some of the best and eventually some of the worst AIDS coverage in the country, head- lined antigay violence in an article entitled "The West Street Massacre." On November 19, 1980, a 39-year-old former Transit police officer named Ronald Crumpley had opened fire with an automatic weapon in front of the Ramrod bar, located at the farthest end of the West Village and described as "the butchest bar in Manhattan," leaving two dead and several others wounded. The attacker offered that he would have killed more had he not been quite so angry. In part because Ronald Reagan had just beaten Jimmy Carter (with the help of Rev. Jerry Falwell) in the presidential election, in part because Crumpley's father was a minister, publisher Charles Ortleb asked, "Has the Moral Majority sent its first commando into the gay community?"[1]

For many, the profile of the attacker—an ex-cop with a strict reli- gious background—was uncannily similar to that of Dan White, the San Franciscan who had murdered gay activist Harvey Milk and Mayor George Moscone two years before. On the Monday following the Ramrod attack at the second of two memorial marches, the crowd walked from Sheridan Square down Christopher Street to the site of the bar near the Hudson River, where participants sang the venerable American anthem of apoca- lyptic war, "The Battle Hymn of the Republic." In the attack New York's gay men had been assaulted symbolically as well as physically insofar as Marlboro-man styled "clones," a repudiation of "pansy" stereotypes, had been victimized on their own home turf. Three years later, in an advertisement in the same paper, the newly formed National Gay Task Force would caution in large bold type: "They're out to kill! If you are gay or lesbian, you are the target for right wing political opportunists and religious fanatics."

The configuring of this crisis as a war, and not just any war but the ultimate war won by engaging in the final battle, is a characteristically American construction employed at decisive historical moments. It is ultimately derived from the Christian scriptures' notion of Armageddon, the ultimate battle of good and evil represented in the Book of Revelation. This trope, predicated on a demonic Other, has endured in American civic discourse from its beginnings and continued to be not only a pervasive but also a pernicious figure in AIDS politics, pernicious because as Susan Sontag asserted, a military trope "overmobilizes, . . . overdescribes, and . . . powerfully contributes to the excommunicating and stigmatizing of the ill."[2] I will argue in this chapter that military metaphors around AIDS have produced more harm than benefit insofar as they have created false "alliances," produced unrealistic expectations of "victory," and erased subtle political and epidemiological nuances.

The term "Armageddon" appears in the last book of the Christian Bible, the Book of Revelation, where it refers literally to the location of a consummate battle of good and evil on the Plain of Meggido. In the intervening centuries the term has come to apply to any battle or military campaign so configured, such as the Christian apocalyptic crusades against the Islamic nations whom popes and preachers characterized as the Antichrist. With the curious semantic slippage of meaning one typically finds in apocalyptic discourse, "Armageddon" in the late twentieth century has come to be associated with nuclear annihilation, ecological catastrophe, the threat of wayward asteroids striking the earth, and apocalypse itself.

In some of the earliest Anglo-American discourse, Puritans described a millennialist "errand into the wilderness" that required violent struggles against the forces of evil in North America, variously identified as Native Americans (whom some thought to be lost tribes of Israel) or religious dissenters and antinomians (who were characterized as nothing less than Satanists) or French Canadians (whose papist credentials secured their claims to Antichristdom) or eventually in the eighteenth century, the British king. It was this last identification of the Antichrist—the physical, human incarnation of evil or Satan—that energized some of the millennialism of the American Revolution. Midway in the next century,

Americans on both sides of the Mason-Dixon line interpreted their conflicts over slavery as an apocalyptic struggle, prompting Julia Ward Howe's famous anthem, based on the Book of Revelation. One can well ask if the conflict produced the trope or vice versa.

During the 1980s, President Ronald Reagan's initiatives to raise the ante in the Cold War arms race with the Soviet Union (which he configured as an "Evil Empire") promoted widespread scenarios of doom not unlike those of the first nuclear-age decade of the 1950s. Apocalyptic war has been figured in less obviously militaristic contexts. In the United States, periods of social change are often construed as crises, and the responses to these crises are often configured as war: thus we "declare war" on drugs, on crime, on inflation, on terrorism, and on AIDS. As Ernest Tuveson noted, "When urgent and baffling questions about the right course for the nation have arisen, the apocalyptic view of its history has come to the front: at such times as the expansionist eras, the Civil War, the First World War."[3]

AIDS and Military Metaphors

While the figure of Armageddon and its critique have produced a discursive bounty, I am claiming a distinctive reading in the context of a pervasive American apocalyptic language. In this chapter particularly I will explore the apocalyptic significations of AIDS and of queer activist groups in New York, especially ACT UP, and of one activist in particular, journalist and novelist Sarah Schulman, whose activism has also been related to the direct-action group, Lesbian Avengers. I will show how military tropes are initially mobilizing but eventually exhausting, in part because those tropes invent a fictional unity deployed against a demonized opposition, belying the intended subversive use of this dominant discursive form by marginal groups.

Military tropes attached to AIDS are profuse, informing the way we talk about HIV, the body's immune system, sexual dissidents, ethnic minorities and the poor, and the public health system. The trope is evident, for instance, in biomedical discourse; an article in *Poz* magazine, a national bimonthly marketed to HIV positive readers, described "the AIDS battle" as "a titanic struggle in which a crafty and relentless foe eventually wears down the marshaled forces of the immune system, with billions of casualties on both sides each day before HIV ultimately triumphs." New Yorker John Lauritsen similarly configured his collection of AIDS-dissident writing as *The AIDS War: Propaganda, Profiteering and Genocide from the Medical-Industrial Complex*, with the rationale that "[i]n the course of this book it will become plain why I have employed the metaphor of war: the terrible suffering and loss of life, propaganda, censorship, rumors, hysteria, profiteering, espionage, and sabotage." The martial trope has also come to define the ways in which literature about AIDS is received. Living in New York at the time, Andrew Holleran represented the city in the terms of strategic nuclear bombing as "Ground Zero," and wrote, "because as long as it lasts, we must think of it as a war and not some fatal flu, writing about AIDS will appear, and in the short terms will almost inevitably be judged, I suspect, as writing published in wartime is: by its effect on the people fighting. Indeed, it must be about fighting—it must be in some way heartening—it must improve morale, for it to be allowed a place of honor," thus formulating not only a rhetorical trope but identifying a canon of criticism as well: aesthetic production as political utility.[4]

Military metaphors about AIDS have a way of "penetrating" discursive boundaries to attach themselves to other issues as Scott Tucker observed:

> However we choose to conceive of cellular relations, the bodies of women, workers, people of color, queers, people with AIDS, and the disabled are already sites of struggle, including industrial illness and injuries, racial assaults, rape and domestic abuse, queerbashing, and other kinds of physical denial and destruction. In the debates over gays in the military, there was much concern that whole battalions would be emasculated by the mere glance of a queer, whereas outright gaybashing in and out of uniform is still tolerated as good sport. These are the collateral casualties of the cultural war.[5]

Tucker's manifesto *Fighting Words* attempted to dismantle the constructed boundaries between "private" concerns and "public" concerns in much the same way that AIDS discourse tends generally. Since he was writing a call to action, his employment of the tropes of war was aimed at mobilizing the left to a strategy.

Such martial tropes have also been the most widely critiqued of AIDS representations. In particular, Susan Sontag was an early critic of military metaphors, acknowledging that while "one cannot think without metaphors . . . that does not mean there aren't some metaphors we might

well abstain from or try to retire."[6] She summarized a Western genealogy
of medical tropes, observing that the military figures came into widespread use during World War I and contended that by constructing a
demonic "enemy," military medical tropes fashion "innocent victims,"
leading inexorably to stigmatizing the "guilty." In *Illness as Metaphor*, her
first meditation on illness specifically derived from her own experience of
cancer, Sontag had contended that some metaphors kill and had asserted
that her project was to render the disease "meaningless," that is, as just
a (very serious) disease with no implications of guilt or shame. However,
she pointed out that military tropes of cancer are different from those of
AIDS in their different treatment of the issue of causality. With cancer,
causality is unclear and the body is represented as undergoing a civil war;
with AIDS, causality is clear (at least in her early reading, without benefit
of multifactorial theories) and the body is represented as undergoing an
attack from an alien enemy, thus reproducing the paranoid discourse of
politics, including discussions of the separation or quarantine of the
infected. As Sontag notes in her conclusion to the essay,

> [T]he medical model of the public weal, is probably more dangerous
> and far-reaching in its consequences, since it not only provides a per-
> suasive justification for authoritarian rule but implicitly suggests the
> necessity of state-sponsored repression and violence (the equivalent of
> surgical removal or chemical control of the offending or "unhealthy"
> parts of the body politic). But the effect of the military imagery on
> thinking about sickness and health is far from inconsequential. It
> overmobilizes, it overdescribes, and it powerfully contributes to the
> excommunicating and stigmatizing of the ill.[7]

Brian Patton in "Cell Wars: Military Metaphors and the Crisis of
Authority in the AIDS Epidemic" expanded on Sontag's critique and
associated the seeming "naturalness" or "transparency" of military metaphors with their familiarity, which is also to say, their authority. He
uncovered these flawed tropes in both popular mass discourse (a *National
Geographic* article on the immune system and AIDS) and technical biomedical discourse (a *Scientific American* article by Robert Gallo, an official
"codiscoverer" of HIV). In a postscript to the article, Patton described
Christine Gorman's 1991 *Time* article that configured AIDS and an anti-
AIDS vaccine as high-tech stealth fighter airplanes, technologies then
familiar to Westerners from television coverage of the Persian Gulf War.

However, the technology that could not protect us from HIV in the first place may not so easily save us from it now. The Baby Boom generation initially affected by AIDS had trusted that post-World War II medical technologies (like antibiotics and vaccines) could treat any microbial disease; although AIDS should have disabused us of that notion, we still place our faith in biomedical technologies orginating in the military-industrial complex. Thus coming on the heels of the United States' World War II victories, we were lulled into a trust in technologies. In "AIDS and the American Health Polity: The History and Prospects of a Crisis of Authority," Daniel M. Fox made a similar point, namely that by the 1970s the American consensus that physicians and medicine were generally effective and virtuous had begun to disintegrate. Sarah Schulman also reflected this cynicism in her article "Women Need Not Apply: Institutional Discrimination in AIDS Drug Trials." The exclusion of women from the development of medical therapies would eventually prompt women's militant action in such groups as ACT UP/New York Women and AIDS Book Group and the Lesbian Avengers, both of whom I will discuss later in this chapter.[8]

Less concerned than Sontag with the disvalue of military metaphors, Michael S. Sherry analysed the imaginative and political work they perform. He noticed three categories of imagery: the "war on AIDS" metaphor in dominant discourse; the "holocaust" metaphor in marginal militant discourse; and the representation of casualty in "less overtly polemical genres, especially the descriptive and fictional [writing] that gay male writers compiled in the 1980s." Sherry pointed out that the war metaphors for AIDS were used across the political spectrum, in which different purposes share a common language. He contended that in the antistatist political climate of the 1980s, which was cynical about "big government," employing the language of war legitimated a call for increased federal involvement in AIDS research, treatment, and education, since the military complex is the only form of "big government" that political conservatives seem to countenance. However, he also noted that while military rhetoric has probably served the tactical purpose of mobilizing gay communities, people with AIDS, the government, health professionals and others, it might only have done so at the expense of long-term commitment and participation. The language of war composes a binary resolution of victory or defeat, which oversimplifies the complexities of a medical problem like AIDS. The U.S. experiences in Korea and Vietnam should have demonstrated the American public's distaste for prolonged and uncertain military ventures. Thus Sherry suggested that the language of a " 'war on AIDS' was therefore an ambiguous basis for mobilizing either government or the gay and lesbian community itself . . . that indeed war might be a metaphor of limited utility," a trope of tactical but not strategic usefulness. Sherry made one more point that I find important:

> [T]he political language of AIDS, including that of gay men, has operated more firmly in American political traditions than is usually acknowledged—either by gay militants who trumpet novelty of their tactics or by their opponents who regard them as alien to all that is American. As has usually been the case in American culture, even the novel event had to be translated into language with imaginative sign-posts to the familiar, and even those marginal to the culture must employ—albeit often in atypical ways—its language, assumptions, and methods.[9]

As I have contended throughout this study, queer discourse on AIDS reproduces the binary oppositions and sexual anxieties of the dominant culture, specifically of a Western apocalyptic discourse that predates the modern era. Further, although queer communities may position them-selves as dissident outsiders of a dominant culture, their doing so is precisely within the forms of social and discursive identification articulated in the Protestant Reformation.[10]

AIDS SERVICE ORGANIZATIONS AND MILITANT ACTIVISM

Although Larry Kramer and others frequently gave the impression that no militant AIDS activism existed in New York before they came to-gether in 1987 to form the AIDS Coalition to Unleash Power (ACT UP), there were several grassroots efforts, less well publicized especially in comparison to ACT UP's later successes and with fewer numbers of participants. Reporting in December 1985 in the *New York Native*, Sarah Schulman described the presence of about fifty activists outside New York's City Hall during hearings by the city's Health Committee. Among these was David Summers, a singer/actor and representative of the advo-cacy group People With AIDS, who despite having been invited to testify at the hearings found himself arrested and handcuffed by the police when he tried to cross police lines in order to enter the building, in what

Schulman counts as New York's first arrest for AIDS activism. She noted also that Summers was later joined in this rank by other activists, like Michael Hirsch and Max Navarre, who are often forgotten because "in AIDS politics, he who lives longest, declares history." At this time, lesbians also began to join gay men in AIDS activism, including Maxine Wolfe and Abby Tallmer, since lesbians had been lumped together in the popular mass consciousness with male queers as AIDS carriers (despite most lesbian sex practices being low risk for infection).[11]

Another demonstration on June 27, 1985, at lower Manhattan's Federal Plaza protesting government inaction in the epidemic was organized by Rapid AIDS Mobilization (RAM), a New York-based group whose spokesperson was Buddy Noro. In Noro's press release after the event, he characterized the demonstration as "the beginning of a nationwide movement." And its promotional flyer urged, "This is an overdue call to mobilize! We are literally fighting for our lives!" and also spoke of AIDS as a "political weapon" and a "plague." The calls for mobilization, however, were not very successful, perhaps in part because the activists did not command adequate coalition support or media visibility.[12]

In the summer or fall of 1986, a group calling itself "The Lavender Hill Mob" formed, and by the time its first newsletter was published in January 1987 the group had already challenged the National Conference of Catholic Bishops, then archbishop of New York John J. O'Connor, politicians at the archbishop's annual Alfred E. Smith dinner, editors of the *New York Times*, local radio personality Bob Grant, New York's Senator Alphonse D'Amato, and residents of Howard Beach, actions for which the group had also received media attention. The Lavender Hill Mob encompassed gay rights as well as AIDS issues and members Michael Petrelis, who would eventually become a high-profile national activist, and Marty Robinson met with a New York Food and Drug Administration director in March 1987, the same month ACT UP held its first meeting. In its June 1987 newsletter, The Lavender Hill Mob acknowledged ACT UP's Wall Street and Post Office demonstrations with the comment, "At last some company."[13]

Although New York City will seem to outsiders a paragon of tolerance for diversity, the city is a network of competing social interests usually kept in check by a tenuous political balancing act. Nonetheless, antigay violence is substantial and conservative Christian (Catholic or Protestant) and Jewish religious enclaves are powerful and vocal in their opposition to equal protection for sexual minorities. For example, an article in the *Native* in early 1981 discussed comments by the head of New York's chapter of Moral Majority, who blamed antigay violence on homosexual deviance. Sarah Schulman's two 1985 reports on the hearings of the City Health Committee noted the testimony of one minister:

> Cecil Butler, a Baptist minister and frequent demonstrator in front of St. Mark's Baths, testified for restrictions [of the HIV infected]. "There is an arrogant community within the gay community," he said. "They will not allow you, as a city, to protect its citizens. The gay community doesn't want you to know that there is a smokescreen to cover up the goings-on. They have pedophiles marching in their gay parades; they have sado-masochists." Butler also said that the *Native* was used by men with AIDS to find sex partners.[14]

Another example of indigenous hostility toward gays appeared in an anonymous flier circulated in Brooklyn in the early years of the epidemic that announced:

> A.I.D.S is not caused by Haitians, or by intravenous drug users. It is caused by gays, and by gays alone. By encouraging or protecting the gays we are committing suicide. Gay rights and gay parades will cause the death toll to rise. There is no cure other than to stop the gays. Homosexuality must be outlawed, or else death will spread like wildfire. Take action now. It is already too late.[15]

The last two lines are the most alarming. The anonymous author sounded the usual apocalyptic note, simultaneously urging action while denying human agency. No specific "action" to take was offered, leaving it to the impulses of the reader. These examples indicate the remarkable fluidity of military tropes, which can be employed by competing groups with conflicting politics. When employing military tropes for vastly different political ends, however, the ideological construction is approximately the same: inventing a fictional unity against a demonized enemy. While enclaves of sexual tolerance do exist in New York and the sheer size of the urban population affords sexual dissidents anonymity and safe spaces, they are never far from either militant verbal abuse or physical violence.

Similar to their political opposites, AIDS affected groups employed military figures in order to represent their struggle against the epidemic and against social hostility. Admittedly, early AIDS activism generally entailed advocacy on behalf of the infected or the sick, work that still continues today. The activism of Gay Men's Health Crisis (GMHC), People With AIDS Coalition, Harlem's Upper Room shelter for the homeless with AIDS, AIDS Treatment Data Network, Housing Works, and others, was not militant, but attempted to work within existing social structures in the space opened up by more vocal critics like Larry Kramer. However, AIDS service organizations have used militaristic rhetoric to promote fundraising efforts, similar to the NGTF lobbying advertisement noted above.

The Human Rights Campaign Fund (HRCF—now known as Human Rights Campaign), for example, in a 1983 advertisement allied with GMHC to promote a joint fundraising rodeo, proclaiming "Join the Two-Front War on AIDS." Although HRCF's aims have always been explicitly political ("Keeping your friends in Congress—and your enemies out" the ad's motto announces), this collaborative effort with GMHC proposed an "all-out war on AIDS" in a "joint assault on the common enemy: AIDS." Thus the advertisement seems confused about the identification of the enemy (Is it AIDS? Is it certain socially conservative politicians? Is it both?), a strategic flaw in much queer politics. HRCF's ad proposed that it and GMHC were jointly "marshalling the resources of the community to protect the healthy and nurse our fallen" as well as "defending our community and helping to lead the battle against AIDS."

This rhetorical excess reflected the extreme anxiety, especially in New York, as gay men in particular entered the third year of the announced epidemic, but it also exemplified some of the strategic hazards in using martial tropes. First, as noted, there needs to be an enemy, thus tactically constructing an oppositional politics that may not always be strategically effective; and if the ideological agenda becomes too complicated, a "campaign" may be opened on too many "fronts" at one time. Furthermore, an "all-out war" precludes compromise and concession, which will always be a political reality. Second, a declaration of war is usually accompanied by the obliteration of internal differences and the affirmation of an imagined "unity" in the name of a fictive, homogenous "nation"; thus the advertisement refers to "our friends," "our fallen," and "our community," though the interests of an HIV infected female drug user in Harlem may be conspicuously different from those of a gay male investment banker in the West Village. Not to mention that the fund raiser's $200 ticket price would probably exclude the first. While the AIDS epidemic has revealed New York's numerous social and economic differences, similar language would still be employed. For example, in 1995 the Housing Works Theatre Project, an advocate for homeless people living with AIDS, produced *Burned Out City*, a fundraising musical written and performed by its clients. Advertising copy for the performances read: "When the war has taken its toll get ready for *Burned Out City*."

Act Up

As the decade of the eighties wore on, Larry Kramer and others began to call for more militant action, not simply on behalf of the sick or the dying, but to stimulate institutional action on treatments and a cure for AIDS. When Kramer was asked to replace a last-minute cancellation of guest speaker Nora Ephron at the Lesbian and Gay Community Services Center on March 10, 1987, a certain "critical mass" had accumulated so that his call for a new kind of activism produced subsequent meetings that resulted in the formation of ACT UP.

The group wasted no time. Its first action, No More Business as Usual, a demonstration on Wall Street aimed at drug companies' "profiteering" (itself a term carrying wartime connotations) was held later that month and resulted in seventeen arrests from among several hundred people participating in the action and eventually produced changes in the Food and Drug Administration's drug approval process, though it would take subsequent actions against drug manufacturers like Burroughs Wellcome to lower the cost of medications. Larry Kramer had published an op-ed piece in the *Times* the day before the demonstration (a bit of careful timing that would have taken some political clout in the newspaper's editorial offices, perhaps shamed by his public excoriation of the paper in *The Normal Heart*) reciting the basic statistics of AIDS and enumerating the demonstrators' demands, information that the group also provided in fact sheets distributed to the business workers who came into contact with the event[16] The group did not spend a great deal of time on organizational issues, and instead, having reached a consensus on the actions, spent its energies and time on planning and implementation of the events. As a result it was able to respond quickly and to draw in a large number of novice volunteer activists whose talents could be engaged immediately, rather than having to confront the inertia that affects most volunteer organizations. ACT UP succeeded in capturing the imagination of many younger gay and lesbian people, some of whom were also artistically creative, adding to the group's erotic appeal and providing collective efforts that produced attention-getting graphics and events. Thus AIDS activism for a while, like antiwar activism two decades prior, became "the scene" for young people where interesting things were happening. This initial success revealed that changing dominant structures often required establishing a momentum through mass media in order to overcome bureaucratic inertia.

ACT UP's media savvy can be demonstrated by several tactics its members employed in order to get the attention of different audiences. Activists knew that in New York, today's wheat-pasted poster will be covered over by a competing advertisement tomorrow; thus "snipers" were hired who would replace posters when they became covered. As a grassroots organization, ACT UP initially did not have the financial resources to secure media attention, so the activists strategized free access opportunities. The No More Business As Usual action targeted the business district for rhetorical as well as thematic purposes: bringing the United States' financial capital to a stop for a few hours promised media coverage. In its second action, ACT UP came to the city's General Post Office late on the evening of April 15, when there were lines of last-minute federal income tax filers, a captive audience for the activists' information sheets on federal AIDS spending. Because the group capitalized on the fact that every local television news program sends a camera and reporter to do a "story" on the late tax-return filers, they guaranteed TV coverage. Wherever there were television or newspaper cameras, ACT UP's adopted logo, the pink triangle on black background with the formula "Silence = Death," was also visible, an implicit elision of the AIDS epidemic with the Nazi's campaign against homosexuals, Jews, Gypsies and other minorities during World War II.

In the concentration camps, internees were required to wear the emblem of their "crime" of incarceration: Jews, two gold triangles forming a star of David; lesbians, a black triangle; homosexual men, a pink triangle; and so forth.[17] Gay activism had employed the recuperated sign of the pink triangle at least since the 1970s. In 1986, an activist collective of six gay men calling themselves the Silence = Death Project produced and "sniped" the poster at their own expense, and attending early ACT UP meetings, donated the design for the new group's post office demonstration. Eventually this design appeared on placards (the posters mounted on foamcore boards), stickers, T-shirts, and buttons, its verbal formula translated into many languages other than English and eventually supple-

mented with the corollary, "ACTION = LIFE." The utter simplicity of
the graphic design constructed a visual version of the political "sound
bite," the emblem and motto reminiscent of Renaissance emblem books
or early American primers. The message was simple and the design,
immediately recognizable.[18] In fine print at the bottom, the first poster's
copy read: "Why is Reagan silent about AIDS? What is really going on at
the Center [sic] for Disease Control, the Federal [sic] Drug Administration,
and the Vatican? Gays and lesbians are not expendable . . . Use your
power . . . Vote . . . Boycott . . . Defend yourselves . . . Turn anger, fear, grief
into action."[19] Thus the activists urged both passive and active resistance to
what they construed as "war crimes" perpetrated by political, governmen-
tal, and religious institutions upon the HIV infected and their friends.

ACT UP explicated this trope of war crimes in an installation called
Let the Record Show, which was situated at the New Museum of Contemporary Art on lower Broadway in the city's artistic "SoHo" section (the
area *South* of *Hou*ston Street, the lower border of Greenwich Village).
The museum's curator, Bill Olander, himself living with an AIDS diagnosis and a member of ACT UP, offered the group the site's display
window for a work on AIDS. An ad hoc collective of artists, designers,
and skilled artisans came together and produced a multimedia installation within a few months. The installation featured large graphics, a neon
version of Silence = Death, and an electronic banner or headline (shades
of Times Square) that documented government inaction with AIDS.
Large stock photographs of Nuremberg war crimes trial defendants
backgrounded contemporary photos and statements by "AIDS crimi-
nals," like those of an anonymous physician ("We used to hate faggots
on an emotional basis. Now we have good reason."), Rev. Jerry Falwell, and
President Ronald Reagan.[20] This ad hoc group decided to continue working as an autonomous collective, calling themselves "Gran Fury" (after the
Plymouth automobile model used by the New York City Police Department), though for a time still associated with ACT UP. Other AIDS-
activist/artist collectives subsequently emerged, including Little Elvis, Wave
Three, and Boy With Arms Akimbo, as well as several video collectives:
Testing the Limits, DIVA TV (Damned Interfering Video Activist Television), and LAPIT (Lesbian Activists Producing Interesting Television).[21]

Understanding a postmodern art context is useful in order to read
the AIDS-related work of activist artists and their use of martial tropes.
Stylistically, the *Let the Record Show* installation would have reminded
those in the art world of the methods of Hans Haacke and Jenny Holzer,

and thus might have seemed too derivative. However, as Douglas Crimp and Adam Rolston point out, "The aesthetic values of the traditional art world are of little consequence to AIDS activists. What counts in activist art is its propaganda effect; stealing the procedures of other artists is part of the plan—if it works we use it." This postmodern activist aesthetic reiterated Andrew Holleran's point quoted earlier that AIDS cultural production must be evaluated by its efficacy, not by purely formal standards. In addition, the mainstream art world was slow to acknowledge AIDS, revealing the distance between the emerging downtown SoHo artists and galleries and the established midtown artists, galleries, and museums. For example, a 1988 exhibit at the Museum of Modern Art (MOMA), entitled "Committed to Print: Social and Political Themes in Recent American Printed Art," failed to include work about gay liberation or the AIDS crisis. The exhibit's curator, Deborah Wye, admitted she knew of no graphic work of artistic quality dealing with AIDS, despite the ubiquity of the Silence = Death posters and the local and national media coverage of ACT UP demonstrations and graphics. In addition, these works were produced by collectives, whose postmodern death-of-the-artist sensibilities subverted traditional notions of artistic production and intellectual property and whose names were not as familiar as those of Rauschenberg, Stella, Haacke, and Kruger who were included in the MOMA exhibit. As Crimp and Rolston pointed out:

> The distance between downtown and uptown is thus figured in more ways than one. . . . Questions of identity, authorship, and audience— and the ways in which all three are constructed through representation—have been central to postmodernist art, theory, and criticism. The significance of so-called appropriation art, in which the artist forgoes the claim to original creation by appropriating already-existing images and objects, has been to show that the "unique individual" is a kind of fiction, that our very selves are socially and historically determined through preexisting image, discourses, and events.[22]

These issues were apparent in the work of individual artists like David Wojnarowicz and Keith Haring, who often appropriated images from other cultural referents and frequently worked gratuitously (for example, Haring's subway art or Wojnarowicz's building wall stenciling). The midtown art world is imbued with an understanding of art as a commodity, an investment that appreciates over time, while the art world's individualism is predicated on the realities of a consumer capitalism that atomizes human collectives into discrete "producers" and "consumers" within "niches" or "markets." This has constructed a "winner-take-all" art market in which a very few artists fetch inflated prices for their work, while the majority are left with little income from theirs.

Activist artists also tend to produce art that people can put to quotidian use, not to venerate as sacred objects in museums and galleries or to inventory among one's assets and investments. In this respect activist art is closer to folk art or to premodern art. Medieval manuscript illuminators, for example, would probably be horrified today to see their pages separated from the books' spines and displayed in picture frames. Crimp and Rolston offered one reading of the work these AIDS graphics perform:

> AIDS activist art is grounded in the accumulated knowledge and political analysis of the AIDS crisis produced collectively by the entire movement. The graphics not only reflect that knowledge, but actively contribute to its articulation as well. They codify concrete, specific issues of importance to the movement as a whole or to particular interests within it. They function as an organizing tool, by conveying, in compressed form, information and political positions to others affected by the epidemic, to onlookers at demonstrations, and to the dominant media. But their primary audience is the movement itself. AIDS activist graphics enunciate AIDS politics to and for all of us in the movement. They suggest slogans (SILENCE = DEATH becomes "We'll never be silent again"), target opponents (the *New York Times*, President Reagan, Cardinal O'Connor), define positions ("All people with AIDS are innocent"), propose actions ("Boycott Burroughs Wellcome").[23]

But aside from any information that the graphics would convey—and as Larry Kramer had come to insist later in his activism, data alone do not mobilize people—these images operated paradoxically within the semiotic regimes of capitalism, in the practices of consumer advertising, activating a mass audience's hunger for solidarity and identification and its identification of solidarity with discrete styles and recognizable insignias. Thus, for example, the Silence = Death T-shirts became a kind of activist uniform—like an army's, such uniforms produce solidarity—eventually joined by a variety of queer-styled shirt graphics, whose most popular brand label was the "Don't Panic" line. Because many AIDS demonstration graphics are visually arresting, employing hip colors and type fonts and frequently ironic postmodern cultural referents, they have also ended up framed on walls of homes where they serve as mementos, memorials, and decoration, as well as conspicuous displays of a status marker. Like wartime propaganda, these graphics staked out one's ideological alliances and served as mementos of past mobilizations or demonstrations.

Three ACT UP demonstration graphics strike me as particularly intriguing uses of the military trope. The first featured a photograph of two World War II sailors locked in an embrace and a kiss with the motto, "READ MY LIPS." (A companion poster featured a photograph of a lesbian couple from a 1920s Broadway play.) Gran Fury prepared this poster for Nine Days of Protest, the first nationally coordinated AIDS demonstrations, which included "kiss-ins" by gays and lesbians emphasizing that erotic connections were still possible during the epidemic. While sailors have long provided images of desire in homoerotic art, these two figures subverted the conventional image in which the sailor is the subject who gazes or the untouched object of another spectator's gaze, by instead turning to another sailor in physical intimacy. This image and the disturbing resonances it produced for heterosexuals would become a salient four years later in the debate over gays in the military.[24]

The second graphic was a crack-and-peel sticker designed by Ken Woodard for the March 28, 1989 Target [New York] City Hall action. About the size and shape of a theatre ticket, the sticker is divided into two halves. The top half reproduced an explicitly militant ACT UP chant, "ACT UP, FIGHT BACK, FIGHT AIDS," before giving the date and time of the event. In the lower half red letters ringed a red bull's eye: "TARGET CITY HALL." ACT UP's explicit goal in this demonstration was for the first time to gather large numbers of demonstrators, mobilizing those who had never participated in such actions before. The paradox of this "ticket" to the demonstration was that, unlike usual military practices, organizers revealed their tactics in advance. This was no "surprise attack" or "commando raid" but an attempt to "enlist" or "recruit" new activists, which ended up being quite successful. Although not using the terms "enlist" or "recruit" they are implied in the graphic and provide an ironic subtext in light of the common allegation that homosexuals "recruit" heterosexuals into their "lifestyle."

The third graphic employed the United States' flag, long an emblem of American militarism. Prepared by Richard Deagle, Tom Starace, and Joe Wollin as a subway poster for Independence Day commemorations in 1989, American Flag included standard white stars on a field of blue, but the red stripes are composed of continuously running text: "OUR GOVERNMENT CONTINUES TO IGNORE THE LIVES, DEATHS

AND SUFFERING OF PEOPLE WITH HIV INFECTION BECAUSE THEY ARE GAY, BLACK, HISPANIC OR POOR. BY JULY 4, 1989 OVER 55 THOUSAND WILL BE DEAD. TAKE DIRECT ACTION NOW. FIGHT BACK. FIGHT AIDS." The United States Supreme Court had recently ruled that the desecration of the flag was a constitutionally protected form of free speech, a decision that prompted many politicians to mount soapboxes and introduce legislation to "protect" the flag. Neofascist skinheads in New York took advantage of the controversy to engage in violence.[25] Ironically, the ACT UP "battle call" was not much different from that of the anonymous antigay flier circulated in Brooklyn which similarly admonishes, "Take action now." In both cases, the discourse producers constructed themselves as "threats" to an oppositional "enemy." However, while the discourse was analogous, it was not commensurate: queer adolescents have not forayed into hetero-Christian neighborhoods to assault their residents. Nonetheless, while the rhetoric of alarm is often tactically effective in mobilizing support, it condenses (and thus censors) participants around a pair of polarized positions.

For many young gay men, ACT UP's militarism provided another more gendered function that might otherwise have been missing in their individual histories. Because we often experience ourselves as fundamentally "other" or "different" or "queer" from our fathers and brothers, gay men frequently avoid or are deprived of rituals of male initiation into sexuality, courage, aggression, competition, and physical competence. As Tim Miller remarked, ACT UP had a highly military ethos, including its own stylized (and stylish) "uniform," and "medals" that incorporated many elements of male initiation. In fact, he contended, ACT UP was "better at warrior initiation than political action." However, this initiation was useful, Miller suggested, for young men facing death (their own or others') who often had been "colonized by their fathers." What is interesting about Miller's reading of ACT UP is his enculturated placement of males in the role of warrior, although the women's Lesbian Avengers would also configure themselves as warriors.[26]

LESBIAN AVENGERS

Like an earlier activist precursor, Gay Men's Health Crisis (GMHC), Lesbian Avengers began in someone's living room. In the spring of 1992, however, the concerns were women's health and lesbian visibility.

Anne-Christine D'Adesky, Maxine Wolfe, Marie Honan, Ann MaGuire, Sarah Schulman, and Ana Maria Simo gathered in Simo's apartment to discuss the formation of a lesbian direct-action group. They decided on an action on the first day of school in Queens District 24, whose school board had been leading the effort to defeat a proposed multicultural curriculum (which included sexual minority awareness). Planning and recruiting for the action took place over the summer, including the group's distributing 8,000 "club cards" announcing "WE WANT REVENGE AND WE WANT IT NOW!" and inviting interested lesbians to a July meeting at the Lesbian and Gay Community Services Center. Later that fall, about fifty Lesbian Avengers gathered outside a working-class Middle Village Queens schoolyard to chant and distribute lavender helium filled balloons with the motto: "Ask About Lesbian Lives." Many parents accompanying the children forbade them from accepting the balloons while others let their children keep them; but insofar as all the children and their parents heard the word "lesbian" and had to discuss it with their children, the action was a success. As Sarah Schulman pointed out, this action became characteristic of the Avengers' work:

> We were willing to confront the greatest taboo in the culture—homosexuals in the school yard. And we did it in a creative, imaginative, and constructive way. It was a strong, radical, confrontational action. But it was friendly. It also set a pattern for our future of going directly to the sources that are attacking us and confronting them on their territory. This was a big step for the lesbian movement, away from symbolic actions or safe, comfortable critiques of other liberal organizations. It focused our work directly on the right wing, and established a new tone for lesbian politics—a post-ACT UP lesbian movement.[27]

In that final characterization, Schulman was both giving credit to and prefiguring the decline of the earlier AIDS activist group.

An early promotional handout for Lesbian Avengers captured the discursive flavor of the organization. Printed on 22 x 34 inch newsprint and employing various type fonts and sizes, the headline announced, "DYKE MANIFESTO. CALLING ALL LESBIANS! WAKE UP!" while a footer asserted, "The Lesbian Avengers. We Recruit," playing ironically on the right-wing hysteria that maintains that queers are made, not born. The manifesto continued:

It's time to organize and incite. It's time to get together and fight. . . . It's time for a fierce lesbian movement and that's *you*: the role model, the vision, the desire. WE NEED YOU. Because: we're not waiting for the rapture. We are the apocalypse. We'll be your dream and their nightmare.

The manifesto is, of course, explicitly millenarian. "Rapture" adverts to a fundamentalist belief formulated in the nineteenth century that the elect will be taken up into heaven before Armageddon. In claiming themselves as apocalyptic, Lesbian Avengers followed an ancient Western Christian formulation: the eschaton will reveal good news for Us, bad news for Them. Further down, in the "below the fold" section of the publication, the manifesto asserted, "Lesbian Avengers . . . believe direct action is a kick in the face . . . plan to target homophobes of every stripe and infiltrate the Christian right." The bottom of the sheet featured the group's logo, designed by Ana Maria Simo's son Thomas, a cartoon ball-shaped bomb with a lit fuse, which would be construed by some right-wing partisans as an assertion of anarchistic violence or terrorism.[28]

A signature ritual of the group was fire eating. Choreographer Jennifer Monson had taught Lesbian Avengers the technique used by street and carnival performers, which leant both a subversive cachet and a clear demonstration of the group's militant assertiveness. The ritual included a text as well as the symbolic action:

We take the fire of action into our hearts, and we take it into our bodies, and we stand here and now to make it known that we are here and here we will stay. Our fear does not consume us. Their fire will not consume us. We take that fire and we make it our own.

This ritual was simultaneously directed at an outside audience as an intimidating gesture of strength as well as among the members of Lesbian Avengers, for whom it ritualized a militant initiation, which is typically even less available to young lesbians than it is to young gay men.[29]

Over the next two years, Lesbian Avengers continued its actions both in New York City and elsewhere in the country, for which it received some media attention. Probably its most visible event was the co-organizing of a "Dyke March to the White House" in April 1993, the weekend of the nationally organized March on Washington for Lesbian, Gay and Bi Equal Rights Liberation. Lesbian Avengers estimated that 20,000 people marched on the night before the national march. As one participant related, "Just before the march started I turned around and behind me I just saw a sea of lesbians; it was an incredible sight. We just set off down the road; it was like going to Oz." This event created a national network that was employed a few months afterward in response to an HIV-positive lesbian, Dee DeBerry, in Tampa, Florida, who had received threats and whose trailer had been the target of arson while she was in Washington, DC, for the march. Converging on Tampa from New York and elsewhere, Lesbian Avengers made the woman's plight high-profile news, prompting a television appearance by the mayor speaking out against hate crimes. Later in the spring and early summer, the U.S. Congress would hold televised hearings on President Clinton's proposal to permit openly gay or lesbian people into military service. Between those hearings—a painful combination of gay visibility and misrepresentation—and the march, grassroots organizations discovered a growing constituency for activist participation. By 1994, Lesbian Avengers would count thirty-five chapters nationally. This success was partly the result of national recruiting by the journalist, novelist, and activist who had been writing about AIDS activism in New York, Sarah Schulman.[30]

Sarah Schulman: Fiction, Journalism, and Activism

In the late winter and spring of 1993 while on a book tour to promote her fifth novel, *Empathy*, Sarah Schulman crisscrossed the country like an evangelist, fostering Lesbian Avengers chapters wherever she appeared. During the previous decade this native New Yorker had published numerous articles in local and national periodicals. Her first journalist assignment in 1979 when she was twenty-two was for the feminist newspaper, *Womanews*. During the first decade and a half of the AIDS epidemic she also wrote frequently for the *New York Native* and for the *Village Voice*, while also appearing in the *Nation, Interview, Cineaste*, and the *Guardian* of London. In addition, she has published three AIDS-related novels: *People in Trouble, Empathy*, and *Rat Bohemia*.[31] Drawn from her own life, many of her characters inhabit the funky neighborhoods of the East Village and Lower East Side with their heritage of immigrant life, leftist politics, and bohemian poverty, a world she lovingly maps in "When We Were Very Young: A Walking Tour through Radical Jewish Women's History on the Lower East Side, 1879–1919" (*History*, 125–48). Her fiction prose style is intended as a guerilla tactic in an undeclared war over the politic body. In this last section I will discuss two of Schulman's novels dealing with AIDS: *People in Trouble* and *Rat Bohemia*.

About the period in her life that produced Schulman's fourth novel, *People in Trouble*, she has written in "Preface: My Life as an American Artist":

> Continued to write plays. Stayed in ACT UP. Started to experience death of the young on a regular basis. Felt helpless. Saw how alone we are. Lived with dying, participated in denial, felt uncontainable grief. Learned to contain my grief. Wrote on social aspects of AIDS. Grew angrier and angrier at the passivity of artists when it came to politics. Began to hate the avant-garde. Got more involved in ACT UP. Realized that personal homophobia becomes societal neglect. That there is a direct relationship between the two. Wrote a social realist novel *People in Trouble* trying to explain this idea. Tried increasingly to close the gap between politics and art. Could not believe how sexist gay men were. . . . Got arrested with ACT UP when we occupied Grand Central Station at the Day of Desperation Action three days after the beginning of the Persian Gulf War. Wrote more articles about AIDS. (*History,* xviii)

The fragmentary writing condenses a varied emotional and cultural landscape while at the same time it resists the appearance of a flawless or seamless narrative. It also reflects Schulman's ideological commitments to a progressive politics as much as it represents her own conflicted relationship with liberalism and the radical left.

Despite Schulman's own characterization, I am not sure that *People in Trouble* is a social realist fiction, though this may be genre quibbling on my part. Set in New York City, largely in the East Village, the novel features a romantic triangle between Kate, a visual artist with a developing career, her husband Peter, who is a theatrical lighting designer, and her lover Molly, a lesbian and AIDS activist involved in a direct-action group called "Justice," modeled after ACT UP. Throughout the novel, Kate resists immersion in a lesbian identity as she resists surrendering herself emotionally to Molly; she is what might be more accurately described as "queer" in the sense that her marriage to Peter and her affair with Molly respond to her polymorphous desires. However, increasingly Kate is drawn into AIDS activism, which culminates in a fiery apocalyptic conclusion. Schulman wrote both women with passion and tenderness, while Peter (and other men) seem, at least in this male's (perhaps self-absorbed) reading, stereotypical in their self-absorption.

In addition to being a novel about romances (lesbian and heterosexually married), *People in Trouble* is also a social satire, which Schulman seems to intend as social realism. More of the plot's energy concerns the depredations of real estate developer Ronald Horne (shades of Donald Trump). Horne has filled in the lower Manhattan river bank to form "Downtown City," a development for the wealthy. In addition, the land baron has developed a midtown hotel complex called "Castle" which was:

> . . . the biggest, lushest, most ostentatious and expensive hotel from the Eastern Seaboard to Rodeo Drive. . . . It was renowned, not only for its lavishness, but also for the transplanted tropical rain forest that had been re-created inside the lobby to serve as a symbolic moat with actual crocodiles. The guests could feel like authentic aristocracy instead of the robber barons that they really were. From the moment they checked in they were treated like royalty from the middle ages. The motif was Early Modern Colonialism and the staff was required to dress in loincloths with chains hanging from their wrists and ankles. The men's room didn't say Men on the door. It said Bwana. The bathrooms were designed to look like diamond mines with black attendants wearing lanterns and pulling paper towels out with pickaxes. Chicken salad on rye cost twelve dollars. (119)

Horne is also managing to buy downtown apartment buildings with a large number of gay male tenants, speculating that the apartments will become available for condominium conversion as the men die from AIDS. Drawn into the direct-action group Justice by Molly, Kate participates in her first action when the activists "invade" Horne's Castle. Kate has been invited to produce a public installation, which she calls "People in Trouble" intended as a response to the AIDS epidemic. What she only later discovers is that the site for the installation is another Horne project. When the funeral mourners of a friend who died of complications from AIDS leave the church and march to the Horne site, a riot ensues, ending in the "accident" that kills Horne, caused, the novel implies, when Kate scrambles under the dedication stage and ignites the polyurethane material she has used for the installation. Ironically, Kate's artistic career takes off, and she is commissioned to produce incendiary installations in Europe and the United States. Horne's estate, we are told, is then "purchased by the president of a major chemical company who was himself assassinated by a man dying of cancer" (226). At the end of the novel, one activist admits, " 'Suffering can be stopped . . . [b]ut it can never be avenged, so survivors watch television.' " Even though fantasies of vengeance are typical militant responses to the social conditions around AIDS, they can only remain fantasies.

In a talk presented at the first OutWrite National Lesbian and Gay Writers' Conference in 1990, "AIDS and the Responsibility of the Writer," Schulman repudiated both objectivity and conclusiveness in writing about the epidemic. Having just published *People in Trouble* she recounted the work required for her to write the novel: composing a lexicon or vocabulary, noting details of life under this crisis, constructing characters "to express a precise political idea—namely, how personal homophobia becomes societal neglect" (*History*, 195). In that process, she observed that "just as literature has distorted women into the virgin/whore dichotomy, straight men have been distorted into the hero/villain dichotomy" (*History*, 195), precisely a resistance to a demonizing binarism that martial metaphors require. Schulman also insisted in this talk that:

> Reading a book may help someone decide to take action, but it is not the same thing as taking action. The responsibility of every writer is to take their place in the vibrant, activist movements with everybody else. The image created by the male intellectual model of an enlightened elite who claim that its artwork *is* its political work is parasitic and useless for us. At the same time I don't think that any writer must write about any specific topic or in any specific way—writers have to be free of formal and political constraints in their work so that the community can grow in many directions. But, when they're finished with their work, they need to be at demonstrations, licking envelopes and putting their bodies on the line with everybody else. (*History*, 196–97)

Schulman's insistence that a writer's topics or forms of writing about AIDS do not need to be ideologically prescribed (or proscribed) may have been a response to Edmund White's 1987 *Artforum* article, "Esthetics and Loss," in which White insisted that AIDS writings "must begin in tact, avoid humor, and end in anger."[32] Some of Schulman's disillusionment with avant garde artists in this respect was evident in her essay "Is the NEA Good for Gay Art?" in which she asserted regarding the NEA funding controversies:

> When Cindy Carr said in a second article that she "may now be forced to conceive of a new demimonde—a bohemia of the unfundable," I got really angry. Doesn't she know that 99 percent of the artists in this

country already live in the world of the unfundable? And that this
invisibility is due, in part, to the role played by critics like her? . . . While
we must support lesbian and gay arts, we must also refuse the distor-
tion of calling it "censorship" of the rewarded, while ignoring the thou-
sands who are systematically excluded from support because they don't
fit the profile for privilege. Every out gay artist loses grants, gigs, and
opportunities and faces bias and limitations throughout his or her
career for being gay. This needs to be addressed politically with a
recognition of how homophobia works on all levels, not only in the
case of the most visible. (*History,* 201)

Thus she debunked the fantasy of many artists (and academic critics as
well) that aesthetic or critical production by itself causes social reform.

Additionally, Schulman resisted a sentimentality that constructs the
experience of AIDS as transformative. Sentimental fictions of "family"
are first in her critique. As she noted in a talk given at the 1992
OutWrite conference, "By ignoring our lack of rights and continuing
to exercise theirs, our families are participating in the construction of
a fake life" (*History,* 236). For example, the character of Peter in *People
in Trouble* is not heartless; he just doesn't understand what the fuss is
all about. He is a creature of America's heteronormative culture that
canonizes the nuclear family so that what does not affect him directly
lacks significance. In contrast, the lesbian and gay relationships of the
novel are articulated among lovers, exlovers, and others who construct
extended families of affiliation, not of birth or marriage. The birth-
families of gay men living with AIDS may likewise not be cruel, but
because their experience of "family" is so atomized their compassion
(and their action) cannot extend beyond the "family circle." This issue
would become even more evident in Schulman's later novel, *Rat Bohemia.*
Schulman observed that, "Unfortunately we have constructed expectations for AIDS literature based on this myth of transformation. By
holding it to a standard based on the model of religious conversion, we
expect AIDS literature to reveal profound insights into life and death
that people without terminal illness would not be able to conjure up on
their own. But in reality, the opposite is true" (*History,* 237). In other
words, AIDS only makes us more of what we were before diagnosis. In
this respect, Schulman again resisted the apocalyptic trajectory in which
those who survive Armageddon become the saints—with all the rights
and privileges, like wisdom, pertaining thereunto. What follows Armageddon? Shortly I will turn to her later post-apocalyptic novel to exam-

ine that question. In *People in Trouble* she seemed to say that life for some simply goes on, to other romances and careers. "Then everyone went to Saint Vincent's [Hospital]" Schulman wrote in the novel's last line, "because there was nothing more to say" (228).

Is there hope after Armageddon? And if there is, what grounds it? The conclusion to *People in Trouble* seems cynical in some respects. Kate's presumed spontaneously transgressive act of setting on fire her installation—and with it the predatory Ronald Horne—is commodified into an avant-garde formal innovation and her heroism is leveraged into an upwardly mobile career move when she becomes the subject of essays by Gary Indiana in the *Village Voice* and Barbara Kruger in *Artforum*. However, Molly and her activist family continue their direct action. The question of hope is central for understanding Sarah Schulman's fiction, but not simply to register how she appropriates or resists American apocalypticism. In an essay first published in 1991, "Why I Fear the Future," she stated:

> [K]nowing that no large social gains can be won in this period, I still remain politically active. I do this because small victories are meaningful in individual lives. I do this because I don't want to be complicit with a future in which people in need will die and everyone else will be condemned to a vicious banality. But also because I believe that in long, hard struggles, there is a value to what Gary Indiana calls "the politics of repetition." Even if it takes all of our energy, I still intend to do everything I can do to at least keep these issues alive. (*History*, 222)

In a talk presented the next year, "Why I'm Not a Revolutionary," Schulman would note that, "In the vocabulary of the old left, the reason for living was revolution. In our time, however, we comprise the first generation who does not think that the future will be better. We fear the future. We live in a profound state of nostalgia" (*History*, 258). Since revolutionary change is not achievable, Schulman asserted that the concept of *resistance* provides the necessary psychic and ideological structure that makes action possible. And in the queer resistance movements today, "imagination is our secret weapon" (*History*, 239).

People in Trouble has enjoyed a troubled half life in an artistic controversy about plagiarism and straight appropriations of AIDS and gay representations. In 1996, composer/lyricist Jonathan Larson prepared for the premier of his AIDS-themed version of Puccini's *La Bohème*, entitled *Rent*, but died suddenly before its opening night at the New York Theatre

Workshop in the East Village. A rock musical about struggling East Village artists, some of whom are fatally ill, *Rent* uncannily paralleled the life of its creator (who died of the less romantic heart disease than *Rent's* postmodern consumption, AIDS). Larson's untimely death, the show's topical subject, and its frank treatment of sex, drugs, and New York real estate politics, as well as the energy, lyricism, and ingenuity of its music, made it a sensation and it quickly moved to Broadway (and eventually on to a national tour, a Pulitzer prize and Tony Awards). However, for Sarah Schulman, sent to review the production, the musical's plot too closely resembled that of *People in Trouble*. She discerned that the straight elements of the plot came from Puccini but its queer plot came from her novel. However, Schulman's claiming copyright infringement and seeking legal redress was problematic in the face of Larson's apotheosis (he died for his art in the popular perception) and the enormous financial success of the show. Besides, it is less easy to claim plots as intellectual property than it is words. Instead, Schulman wrote her account of the controversy, *Stage Struck: Theater, AIDS, and the Marketing of Gay America*, in which she developed an analysis of the ways in which mainstream dramatizations of AIDS and queer life were pasteurized for the consumption of larger audiences, such as Larson's sentimentalization of East Village "bohemian" life.[33]

Sarah Schulman's more recent AIDS-themed novel, *Rat Bohemia*, is also her most fully realized. If her earlier AIDS novel was raw and polemical, this one is wiser and more compassionate, like Larry Kramer's movement from harsh didacticism in *The Normal Heart* to a greater human sympathy and forgiveness in *The Destiny of Me*. Set again in the East Village, *Rat Bohemia* concerns three friends: Rita Mae Weeks, a rat exterminator for the city; her friend David, a gay writer with HIV; and her woman friend Killer, a career plant waterer. This trio is joined by others, notably by Killer's new girlfriend, Troy, and by the established but closeted lesbian writer, Muriel Kay Starr, whose four chapters from a novel called *Good and Bad* comprise the concluding appendix to Schulman's novel. The sections of *Rat Bohemia*, several chapters in length, are written as first-person narratives by the three central characters, which provides Schulman the opportunity to produce not only different points of view of the same landscape but also the sounds of different voices. They include anecdotes and vignettes without a unified plot, climax, or resolution.

The East Village locale of this novel seems post-apocalyptic, littered with human and technological remains, a waste heap of history on which the eponymous vermin cavort. Like Melville's cetology, this novel includes considerable *rattus* lore, the vermin becoming symbols of both parasitism and survival. In the book's first section, "Rat Bohemia," Rita offers her technical expertise in rat extermination while narrating the life of her family: her deceased mother a survivor of the holocaust, her adolescent love affair with another girl in the family's apartment building, a relationship that is transformed dramatically when her father walks in on their lovemaking. She concedes the difficulty of being a friend to David, who is narcissistic and self-absorbed, a character defect common to Schulman's male characters, though David at least, unlike Peter of *People in Trouble*, has an AIDS diagnosis to justify it. Rita observes, and here Schulman's own voice from the 1992 OutWrite Conference emerged clearly, that "AIDS is not a transforming experience" and that it has no spiritual message or anything redeeming about it.

Throughout the novel, as Edmund White pointed out in his *New York Times* review, Schulman resisted sentimentality, often to great humorous effect as in this exchange between Rita and David's friend Manuel planning David's memorial:

"How are you doing?" I asked Manuel quickly.

"I am very very angry at those PWLOPWA's."

"What's that?"

"People Who Live Off People With AIDS. If this epidemic ever ends, everyone who is still alive will be suddenly unemployed."

"More histrionics?" I asked.

"I think they should change the name of this disease," he said. "From AIDS to AIDA. Only Leontyne Price can do it justice."

. . . Let's face it, David was a Liza Minnelli fag. This was the guy who used to find out where famous people went to Alcoholics Anonymous meetings so he could hold their hands during the serenity prayer. (153)

She further resisted the utopian dream of a "cure": "There is no cure. There are just certain strange combinations of beliefs, acts and events that help some people feel better under some circumstances for some

certain length of time. But there is no way to know why" (53). Having
realized that she will long outlive many of her friends and having dedicated herself to remembering the truth of their lives, Rita concludes the
book's first section by offering her own confession of faith: "[T]he way
I figure it is if I make my contribution to truth, some Rat Bohemian
down the line will notice and appreciate it. She'll be sitting in a city
strewn with rats and rat carcasses and will come across my petite observation. That's the most amazing relationship in the universe. The girl on
rat bones who knows that she is not alone. She is not American" (54).

This conflation of "American" with "lonely" is poignant in the second section, "1984," the year that David, the speaker for much of this
section, believes he was HIV infected. The fact that he engaged in unsafe
sex after the disease and its cause were known occasions David's reflection
on desire and its relation to danger: "Goodness and badness have nothing
to do with it. Desire can't be decided. But there is also that strange
combination of camaraderie in nelly machismo. It is what the literary
critics would call *fabulous realism* if they weren't too stupid to notice"
(58). The year in which Schulman sets this section alludes to George
Orwell's totalitarian dystopia, thus refining the novel's sense of authoritarian threat. "Is getting fucked an act of heroism?" David asks and observes
the culture's bipolar swings between sex and repression: "Apocalypse Now!
Paradise Now! Apocalypse Now! Paradise Now! It's either complete denial
of the virus or complete acceptance" (58–9). What is an obvious allusion
to Francis Ford Coppola's Vietnam-era revision of Joseph Conrad's *Heart
of Darkness* reverberates with the film's and both novels' overwhelming
sense that even military action is pointless, though nonetheless brutally
efficient. What seems to fuel David's rage is a family that carefully manages
its contact and closeness with him, fulfilling the letter of "family values"
without the spirit and blaming him for being different. While acknowledging that his parents were never overtly cruel, he remarks:

> My parents have always hated me for being gay. They've always wished
> I would disappear, but nothing has ever made me so nauseous and
> vicious as the gulf that AIDS has created between me and them. . . . It's
> not AIDS that makes them hate us. They hated us before because they
> could not control us. They could not make us be just like them. Now,
> they're glad we're dying. They're uncomfortable about how they feel but
> really they're relieved. There's nothing on earth that could kill us more
> efficiently than parental indifference. (87)

And when his lover Donny dies from an AIDS-related illness, he assumes the $15,000 cost of the funeral:

> "It's your responsibility," [Manuel] said. "If you ask [his] family for help you'll never forgive yourself." And now I know that he was right. Paying for your lover's funeral is the gay version of a bar mitzvah. It is how you know that you have become a man. (76)

A hell of a way to undergo male initiation. David also recognizes an apocalyptic desire, especially acute for some gay men, that hopes for a male savior. Relating men's reactions at an ACT UP meeting to another activist in the novel, Andrew Barton, David notes: "'We still hope that some male is going to come along and make it all better. But real daddy never did that so why the hell should Prince Andrew?' " (83). For many of us, the eschatological formula, "Some Day My Prince Will Come," is a projection of our own losses and desires, a point that I will expand in the next chapter when discussing the writing of Douglas Sadownick.

The loss and grief of the first two sections are mitigated somewhat by the third, "Killer in Love." Rita's career plant-watering friend, Killer, describes her own struggling relationship with a new girlfriend, Troy, who herself has just ended another relationship: "And all I kept thinking was that I wanted Troy to love me enough that I would never have to speak to my family again" (108). Troy is a poet, who also gets a job in a bakery, and having read the first four chapters of Muriel Starr's *Good and Bad* decides to write a self-help book, *The Millennial Moment: Facing the Coming Millennia* [sic] *with Joy*. In a sketch of the book Troy prescribes eight "leaps of faith" and prophesies, "The old order is rapidly changing. . . . The key to the millennium lies in figuring out what they [the Baby-Boomers] are going to be afraid of. The answer? The future" (118). The future is frightening to most characters in the book. Troy offers an additional prophecy in a conversation with Killer:

> "Future is a scary word here in America," [Troy] said, putting on her spurs. "Americans are dangerous, Killer. We destroy the earth, mind and lymph node and then market that destruction. We make it sound groovy. I have a lot of predictions about the future of America. Predictions that might have already come true."
>
> "Like what?"

"I predict that there will be a new kind of cancer and advertising executives will name it Lymphomania. I predict T-shirts that say *I want to rape you*. I predict haphazard memorial services at every hour of the day and night because too many people are dead. Their ghosts have to compete wildly for remembrance. I predict that homeless people will piss on bank machines like storefronts lined with urinals." (127)

Some of these, of course, have already come to pass.

In the last section, "Rats, Lice and History"—the title pays homage to Hans Zinger's classic 1934 study of plague—Rita's voice returns to narrate David's memorial service, which begins with a march carrying the casket from Houston Street and First Avenue up to Tompkins Square Park. Rita observes that David "wanted his funeral to be the catalyst for the revolution. Who doesn't? And with each AIDS funeral that possibility always lingers. But you can tell within the first ten minutes that it is not going to go that way. People were not furious. Just exhausted" (156–57). After the memorial, Rita finds a bar where the closeted lesbian novelist whose *Good and Bad* almost every character in *Rat Bohemia* has been reading, Muriel Kay Starr, also has come for a drink. Joining Rita, Starr tells her own version of her friendship with David, a revisionist history that Rita questions. The book's third section ends when Rita, her sometime lover Lourdes, Killer and Troy, begin a quickly aborted drive to Delaware to find Rita's first love, Claudia Haas, who is married with children. Rita wonders whether, if she and Claudia hadn't been bullied, they might be the married couple. However, the nostalgic trip is cut short when none of the friends has the cash or credit to fill the gas tank of the rented car, which is returned running on empty.

The book ends with the first four chapters of Muriel Kay Starr's *Good and Bad*. Its title invokes a binary opposition that is foundational to apocalyptic discourse, but its precise significance is ambiguous: The good and bad? The good and the bad? Very bad? Earlier in David's "1984" section, his friend Manuel says, " 'One thing my mother always told me. . . . You'll meet people in your life whose beliefs you despise but they'll be really nice. And then there will be people whose beliefs you embrace but they're awful" (77). Similarly, Schulman refused to demonize even those who had failed her characters the most, their families, even their families of affiliation. As David observes of ACT UP, "It's like a family, I'm telling you. Everyone is too far out of line right in front of each other. I never bring friends to ACT UP. It's like bringing a friend home to dinner when your family is *Who's Afraid of Virginia Woolf?*" (84). Schulman let no one off the hook.

Starr's novel turns out to be a roman á clef, in which Rita is a heterosexual woman, whose father discovers her making love to a young Puerto Rican man and banishes her. She eventually marries David, while Claudia remains the "single career woman," encoding her lesbianism. This conclusion challenges an at-times scorching review of the novel by Vivian Gornick who wrote in *Women's Review of Books*, "The characters in *Rat Bohemia* see themselves as children cast out of Eden; what they want more than anything else is *in*. They want to be enfolded in the embrace of the original family. They want America to love them. That is what they want. They are not bohemians. And I don't think Sarah Schulman knows that."[34] What Gornick missed in her reading is Schulman's obvious ironies, particularly by including the first four chapters of Starr's novel, which demonstrated that even when you want to rewrite the story it still is not going to come out the way you want it; even the fantasy refuses to be idyllic. A short time after David's funeral Rita accidentally meets his father on the street and fantasizes in millenarian fashion:

> Now, I lived in a new world, in a new era. The Post-David Era. And, in the world, those of us who remain can move mountains that the dead could never move. I, Rita Mae Weeks, could convince his father and therefore own his father. Once I transformed his father, his father would belong to me and then, I would have a father. . . . Was this the hidden purpose of AIDS—to give the rest of us a chance to have parents? (199)

Schulman quickly shows us otherwise in her typically desentimentalizing fashion.

Gornick also missed the postmodern irony of "bohemianism," which Schulman clearly understood had become commodified by a late capitalism that uses the ghost of Jack Kerouac to hawk khaki pants for The Gap. " 'So, that was my role in the growth of Queer Nation,' " Troy Ruby tells Killer at one point:

> One minor character in a minor moment. *Queer* did get old very fast, nowadays only academics take it seriously. But *Nation* managed to live on in many fond conversions. Transgender Nation. Alien Nation, Reincar Nation. And all along the line no one noticed how much that word echoed with the secret store of nostalgic desire for normalcy, normalcy,

normalcy. Those apple pie, warm kitchens and American flags that are
trapped somewhere back there between the hypothalamus and the frontal
lobe." (111–12)

Early in the novel, Killer calls contemporary bohemianism "just a state
of mind" and very knowingly explains to Rita the current material conditions necessary for bohemian life:

> In the fifties, the Beats, those guys were so all-American. They could
> sit around and ponder aesthetic questions but a cup of coffee cost a
> nickel. Nowadays, with the economy the way it is, you can't drop out
> or you'll be homeless. You gotta function to be a boho. You have to
> meet the system head-on at least once in a while and that meeting,
> Rita, is very brutal. Nowadays you have to pay a very high price to
> become a bohemian. (30)

Gornick also complaind that the novel's sense of loss, repeated by each
character particularly in relation to family, "must have a clear idea operating behind the sense-impression of unhappiness, guiding and organizing the repetitions. It seems to me that idea is missing in *Rat Bohemia*."
Perhaps Gornick lamented Schulman's refusal to impose a master narrative structuring the characters' losses or she detected Schulman's apparent
relinquishing of a single ideological solution to loss. I would rather suggest that Schulman resisted the "family romance," a kind of millenarian
belief in a past golden age and a future restoration, which each of her
characters falls prey to, and that may be all the idea this book requires.
Far from Gornick's desire for "guiding and organizing," the form of *Rat
Bohemia* meanders, susceptible to the universe's laws of chaos. No critic
of this novel put it quite so well as novelist Edmund White—no stranger
to the literature of AIDS—in his review for the *New York Times*:

> There are few other works of fiction that I could compare with "Rat
> Bohemia . . ." Even her own earlier books, like "People in Trouble" and
> "Empathy," despite the fact that they, too, take place in the East Village
> and deal with AIDS, carry none of the emotional punch of "Rat
> Bohemia." The force of her indignation is savage and has blown the
> traditional novel off its hinges. If she were contributing to the quilt
> project, her quilt would be on fire.[35]

This novel's acutest sense of loss hovers around the eradication of millenarian hope. "[W]e comprise the first generation," Schulman wrote in 1992, "who does not think that the future will be better. We fear the future. We live in a profound state of nostalgia. Concepts like *revolution* just become reminders of the impossibility of change" (*History* 258). Schulman's *idea*, pace Gornick, is that resistance, repeated and daily, remains the only strategy in the current crisis. In both her fiction and her affiliation with Lesbian Avengers, Schulman has demonstrated that militant resistance does not need to be adversarial, although it does need to employ imagination—"[f]or gay people today... our secret weapon" (*History*, 239).

Perhaps the most vigorous critic of martial tropes and calls for militarism has been Schulman's fellow socialist, Scott Tucker, who in a spirited and thoughtful pamphlet has cautioned readers about the tendency for metaphors to become actions. He acknowledged the violence toward gay and lesbian people, against which we have little defense: "Overwhelmingly, straight folks do not know and do not *want* to know the level of violence directed at queers, unless they engage in it themselves." Although the linking of the epidemic with the Holocaust as an analogy "... has some value; as an *equation* it's troublesome." In addition, he rejected queer terrorism:

> For three reasons: Radicals would be idiots to pick general gunfights with the state, since we'd be wildly outgunned and there is *already* bipartisan sentiment to impose a "national security" regime. Also, even if a selective assassination was morally justifiable, like the failed plot to kill Hitler, it is certain that would also involve mass arrests and repression. Finally and crucially, *our movement is ethical and democratic or we are no better than our enemies.*

However, martial tropes in activist discourse are difficult to arrest against an "enemy" that conducts, in its own words, "stealth campaigns" in school board elections; as Tucker asserted, "Politics in this country have been very nasty—indeed, deadly—for many other people, and for a long, long time. Our lives are not negotiable. *Rather than retreat, we fight.*"[36] What is negotiable, to some extent, is the discourse we employ in this struggle, although even that negotiation often seems limited and constrained in a culture where military figures are already naturalized and densely overdetermined. So deeply enculturated, so firmly established and habituated are forms of discourse like these, that they seem to write and read us, rather than the other way around.[37]

Typically, however, the West's apocalyptic trajectory does not end in the devastation of the Battle of Armageddon but imagines a future beyond that conflict. For many people affected by HIV infection and AIDS, the desire for a redemption of suffering has led them to spiritual discourse, often succumbing to its mystifications, but often, too, engaging the ancient problematics of the ideal and real, of the spiritual and the material. In the next chapter I will examine the grounds of post-AIDS hope in the work of two gay Jewish-American writers, playwright Tony Kushner and novelist Douglas Sadownick, and contextualize them in homosexual traditions that imagine bliss through sacred eros. Throughout the AIDS epidemic artists and others have tried to imagine life no longer under this viral sign, often by reconstructing an Arcadian past or by projecting an idyllic future. Whether called "heaven," "cure," "progress," or simply a "future," this imaginary can represent how things might be and thereby mobilize hope.

Chapter Five

Mal'kîm in America

(In memory of Tim)

The Renaissance European imagination violently linked two peoples in such a way that the collision still echoes in American culture, evident in the two AIDS-themed works that are the focus of this chapter, Tony Kushner's *Angels in America: A Gay Fantasia on National Themes* and Douglas Sadownick's *Sacred Lips of the Bronx*. Although in our modern historicist perception the Jewish people and Native Americans could hardly be more distinct from each other, many Renaissance Europeans projected their apocalyptic fantasies on both groups and in some instances even asserted an identity between them.

The year 1492 was catastrophic for both Jews and Native Americans. In Spain, Jewish communities had coexisted with Islamic Moors for centuries in a rich multicultural mixture noted for its textual scholarship and metaphysical reflection. After Ferdinand V and Isabella consolidated their power over the Moors and unified Spain, however, they embarked on a program of "ethnic cleansing" and expelled those Jews who would not convert to Catholicism, in part because Jewish conversion was thought to be a precondition of the Second Coming of Christ. These Sephardic Jews became the bearers of a medieval Jewish mysticism known as Kabbalah (literally, "tradition"), which, as Gershom Scholem argues, took on a markedly different character as a result of their Spanish-imposed diaspora. In that same year, the Spanish monarchs financed a project by an Italian with explicitly apocalyptic aspirations, Christopher Columbus. Columbus believed himself to be a prophet of the End Times and the discovery of a new route to Asia was intended to produce both a treasury of gold and a bounty of souls converted to Catholicism.

Many sixteenth- and seventeenth-century Protestant polemicists reflecting on apocalyptic expectations, which both motivated and were motivated by the Reformation, linked the End Times with the conversion of the Jews while they also employed the Kabbalah's fascination with numerology and alphabetology in their Christian reckonings of the Books of Daniel, Ezekiel, and Revelation. Incredibly to us, some Protestant theologians even identified indigenous Native Americans with the lost tribes of Israel, thus prompting, particularly among the English, proselytizing campaigns in the newly colonized lands. In the nineteenth century this legend of a North American Jewish diaspora would become a part of Mormon mythology, itself an amalgam of Renaissance hermeticism, Judaism, and Christianity. The European colonization of the Americas and the persistent westward advance of Europe's imperial efforts have long been understood as a product of Christian millennialism, specifically the quest for a paradise regained.[1]

In this chapter I will discuss this final apocalyptic trope deployed in the midst of the AIDS epidemic: paradise. For those of the righteous who survive exile or tribulation, the end point of a Judeo-Christian millennialist trajectory is a return to a homeland or a restoration of Edenic bliss, often configured as eternal life in heaven, a mystical union with the Godhead, the Rapture, or even a material millennium, the Reign of God on earth. The Christian Book of Revelation symbolizes this restoration in erotic terms by a marriage of the Lamb (interpreted as Christ) with the Bride (interpreted as the Church or the Elect). If the early AIDS activist Michael Callen attempted to show gay men in New York "How To Have Sex in an Epidemic," later culture workers attempted to show them how to have *hope* in the relentless and ruthless epidemic. Both Tony Kushner's two-part play *Angels in America* and Douglas Sadownick's novel *Sacred Lips of the Bronx* describe the grounds of hope for a post-AIDS queer utopia, inspired by two traditions: hermetic mysticism, particularly Jewish Kabbalah with its emphasis on sacred eros within a complex natural and supernatural cosmology, and a tradition of gay or homo-utopias in the Western literary tradition with its accompanying representation of the erotic sublime. In order to gloss Kushner and Sadownick's work, I will first briefly describe Western hermeticism, then later in the chapter discuss the queer utopian tradition.

HERMETIC MYSTICISMS

"Hermeticism" and "hermetic mysticism" are admittedly problematic terms. They include varied phenomena occurring in diverse cultures over historical periods spanning centuries or even millennia. The name "hermetic" derives from a set of alchemical, occult, or mystical writings composed in Alexandria in about the first century of the Common Era, whose authorship was attributed to the divine Hermes Trismegistus (Thrice-Blessed Hermes). These writings combined Egyptian magic, Jewish mysticism, and Neoplatonic philosophy in tantalizingly obscure language that would engage adherents in the centuries following. One can find their traces in ancient gnosticism and Neoplatonism, medieval Jewish Kabbalah mysticism, Renaissance appropriations and reconfiguration of those traditions in astrology and alchemy, and finally their forms translated to North America, where, among other communities, they found fertile ground in the imaginations of Masons and Mormons. Here admittedly I can only offer a superficial description of phenomena that exist in a variety of forms, each of which is so complex that it could be (and has been) the subject of book-length treatments.

Gnosticism in the ancient world drew adherents among both pagans and early Christians who sought the consolation of mystery religions in order to be freed from this vale of tears. In its first few centuries, the Christian church competed with a variety of Mediterranean mystery religions—communities, texts, and practices that offered eternal life to illuminati by means of gradual initiation into a secret lore about the divine and the material worlds. In some respects this description could include Christianity itself, whose partisans probably objected to gnosticism not because it was so different from Christian orthodoxy but because it was so similar and thus in competition for the same adherents. What we know of gnostic beliefs and practices comes from two sources: a handful of extant contemporary gnostic texts and the more numerous manuscripts of Christian polemicists who refuted them, an admittedly less reliable source. Generally speaking, gnostic beliefs posit a hierarchy of spiritual and material beings, some of whom in varying degrees are declensions from a divine splendor, while others were the work of evil demiurges. The task of the initiate is to overcome this dualism and to ascend by secret or esoteric knowledge (*gnosis*) up toward the divine in order to return to the original splendor by defeating evil. That knowledge was also asserted to have magical powers against the demiurges in the material world, typically in the form of magic formulas. Unlike the Judeo-Christian orthodoxy which imagined an exclusively masculine divinity, gnosticisms also frequently asserted a divine androgyny in which explicitly female attributes were included with the male.[2]

Neoplatonism is derived from ideas in Plato's cosmological *Timaeus*. In a rejection of gnostic dualism, Plotinus, a third-century CE philosopher, posited a divine unity that is the origin of all creation and that creates by means of emanations. Plotinian cosmology found a welcome reception in the early Christian communities, notably in the theological writings of Origen, who by developing the scriptural hermeneutics of the Jewish philosopher Philo of Alexandria appropriated Plotinus in order to develop a theory of the allegorical method of interpreting scriptural texts, and St. Augustine, for whom Neoplatonism provided an alternative to the gnostic and dualistic Manicheism of his youth. Neoplatonism asserts a radical separation of the material and the spiritual world (that is, the world of Ideal Forms), which Christianity complemented with its Christology, the incarnate God mediating between the two orders, thus completing the cosmic hierarchy. Neoplatonic thought has had a remarkably resilient career in Western culture, flourishing during the Middle Ages and Renaissance and again in Romanticism's reaction to Enlightenment materialism and positivism, as well as in some Modernist poetry.[3]

Jewish Kabbalah mysticism draws from both gnosticism and Neoplatonism as well as its own post-Talmudic reflection on the Hebrew Scriptures. It ends where Genesis begins, attempting to describe the inner and precreation or "prehistorical" life of God who is ineffable, a cipher whose mystery resides not in unintelligibility but in "inexhaustible intelligibility." Insofar as it is a midrash or reinterpretation of canonical texts, Kabbalah offers a tradition of continuity; however, insofar as it is a mystical tradition, Kabbalah also makes claims as a prophetic rupture of or supplement to tradition. The classic text of Kabbalah is the thirteenth-century *Zohar* or *Book of Splendor* of Moses ben Shem Tov de Leon, a midrash or commentary on the Torah, which was preceded by the twelfth-century text, *Seper ha-Bahir*, both texts having been developed in Jewish communities of Spain and southern France. While interpreting a canonical text, however, the *Zohar* also proposes its own mythology, including a bigendered divinity, whose contractions and emanations (*Simsum*) formed the created world from him/herself producing the protohuman Adam Kadmon, Kabbalah's androgynous God included female principle,

Shekinah, who was understood to have withdrawn from the male principle in a kind of exile. This divine exile came to be reinterpreted by Sephardic Jews in light of their own expulsion from Spain, particularly in the revision of Kabbalah by Isaac Luria in the sixteenth century. Lurianic Kabbalah was the precursor of a seventeenth-century messianic movement led by Shabbatai Zevi as well as prefiguring an earlier Renaissance formulation of a Christian Kabbalah in Pico della Mirandola and Marsilio Ficino, sources for radical Reformation hermeticisms. While positing a fundamental difference between the divine and the material worlds, Kabbalah mysticism nonetheless urges that everyday life offers access to contemplation and religious ecstasy, nowhere more so than in marital sexual intercourse. Sexuality is understood to unite or restore the ruptured universe, a work produced by every good deed of devout Jews. Kabbalah made two historical entries into American culture: through radical Protestants and later through Orthodox Jewish immigrants.[4]

American Mormonism might even be viewed as a demotic version of Western hermeticism. As John L. Brooke has ably demonstrated in *The Refiner's Fire: The Making of Mormon Cosmology, 1644–1844*, Renaissance hermeticisms were enthusiastically appropriated within radical Reformation traditions and were translated to North America. Particularly in the Early Republic, various groups joined an increasingly complex sectarian mixture in the mid-Atlantic states as antinomian congregations. Brooke notes that:

> The mystical philosophies of alchemy, the Cabala, and more broadly the hermetic theology offered not only a view of the stars but a ladder up through them to the divine Godhead. The goal of hermetic philosophy was to recover the divine power and perfection possessed by Adam before the Fall, and indeed before Creation. Just as the purification of the church by Protestants and Catholics isolated and demonized the cunning folk [Europe's indigenous folk religions' conjurers and witches], so too the hermetic *magus* was expelled in the destruction of the medieval synthesis. When recombined in the Radical Reformation and the English Revolution with currents of millenarian prophecy and a conviction of the imminence of the restored Kingdom of God, hermetic divinization posed a potent challenge to Christian orthodoxy. It also prefigured the cosmology constructed in the 1830s and 1840s by Joseph Smith, who was born in—if not of—a Calvinist culture and moved from the ranks of the cunning folk to the status of an Adamic *magus* as the prophet of the Mormon restoration.[5]

It is precisely this notion of "restoration" that is common to Jewish Kabbalah mysticism and Christian millennialism. Like Kabbalah, Mormonism would claim to be faithful to a tradition while simultaneously claiming a new prophetic vision; and like Kabbalah's historical development in messianic Sabbatianism, Mormonism would tend initially toward an antinomian millenarianism.

Brooke argues that lower New England, along with the upper mid-Atlantic states, far from being a Calvinist hegemony, became the home for numerous sectarian and hermetic groups, whose activities included alchemy, spiritualism, sexual antinomianism, membership in Masonic orders, conjuring, and divining buried treasure. Thus Joseph Smith's ancestral region was saturated with esoteric beliefs and practices that the prophet and founder of Mormonism would "translate" into the angelic discovery of golden plates. Even though the hermetic theology (the Saints' apotheosis into gods) and practices (polygamy) of the Church of Jesus Christ of Latter-Day Saints have modified by means of subsequent revelations since the nineteenth century to come more in line with mainstream Protestantism, Mormonism remains characteristic of what Harold Bloom calls, in an excusable bit of essentialism, the "self-concealed core of the American Religion: Orphic, Gnostic, millenarian."[6]

Jewish mysticism, alchemy (and Jungian appropriations of alchemy), Mormonism, the sacred eros of an androgynous divinity, millennialism, American New Age spirituality: these traditions draw from similar sources, combine in fluid currents, and provide the subtext for Tony Kushner's play cycle, *Angels in America*, and Douglas Sadownick's novel, *Sacred Lips of the Bronx*. In this chapter I will examine the ways in which each writer has constructed from these materials a myth of the erotic sublime that asserts the sacredness of queer sex and that proposes the grounds for millenarian hope in the face of an apocalyptic epidemic.

THE ALCHEMY OF SYMBOLIC CAPITAL: TONY KUSHNER'S *ANGELS IN AMERICA*

Kushner's *Angels in America: A Gay Fantasia on National Themes* (Part One: *Millennium Approaches*, Part Two: *Perestroika*) might be characterized as "fabulous realism."[7] Set in New York, the two plays bring together a WASP with AIDS (Prior) who has been abandoned by his Jewish lover (Louis); their friend, a nurse, who is an Afro-Puerto Rican (Norman

Arriaga, aka "Belize"); a Mormon couple—the husband (Joe) a lawyer protégé of Roy Cohn and the wife (Harper) addicted to Valium; spectral visitations by Prior's ancestors and Ethel Rosenberg, and angels (the Hebrew word is *mal'kîm*). Part One establishes the relationships among these characters, including the preparation of Prior Walter for the first angelic visitation that concludes *Millennium Approaches*. Part Two brings their lives together and anoints Prior as prophet: Louis and Joe briefly become lovers; Harper's alienation from Joe and from reality becomes delusional; Joe's Mormon mother (Hannah) sells her house in Salt Lake City to move to New York City to help the couple; and Belize becomes Roy Cohn's duty nurse as Cohn is dying from AIDS-related illness. Hospitalized himself, Prior is instructed first by a buried text and later by a visit to an angelic council in heaven informing him that God has abandoned the universe because human beings refuse to remain static.

Angels in America has an intricate production history. The plays began with a 1987 commission from Oscar Eustis of San Francisco's Eureka Theater who requested a ninety-minute one-act comedy with music. What he got was a three-act drama, *Millennium Approaches*, which he first workshopped at Los Angeles' Mark Taper Forum in 1990 and premiered at the Eureka a year later. The following January, Declan Donellan directed the play's London production while Eustis and Tony Taccone presented another production at the Mark Taper Forum. The play opened on Broadway in April 1993. Not only was *Millennium Approaches* longer than commissioned, it was also only the first half of a larger work, completed in *Perestroika*. Kushner finished this second play after the death of his mother, whose loss and presence suffuse the piece. This second part was first developed in staged readings at the Eureka in May 1991 and the Mark Taper Forum a year later, where it was premiered in November 1992, opening simultaneously in London and New York a year later. The plays have since been produced in regional and college theaters as well as in a national touring company.

With its length and theatrical effects, *Angels in America* is expensive to produce. By the time of *Perestroika*'s Mark Taper Forum premiere, $1.3 million had already been spent on the production of the two parts. This investment, however, handily paid off: when the Taper box office opened the first day for sales of the double bill, it took in $32,804. This success and that in London brought the plays directly to Broadway instead of moving first to a smaller downtown New York venue.[8] The production values also made the play more accessible to a broader middle-class audience beyond the gay or Jewish theater-goers for whom the play has its most immediate appeal. At a time when gays and "liberals" had become demonized by American conservatives, gay men and progressive Jews were able to see their lives and concerns represented in the main characters of Prior and Louis, as well as in some of the minor characters. According to JoAnne Akalaitis, head of the New York Shakespeare Festival, "What's important about [t]his play is that finally homosexual consciousness, which has been the underground force behind leading art movements in America since World War II, is firmly and visibly out in the center. That's the genius of the project. Tourists from Iowa are going to see it, and it will change culture in America."[9] For an uninitiated audience, the *New York Times* offered a feature on "The Secrets of 'Angels' " in the form of a gloss on some of the plays' arcana. In the two performances of each play that I saw, the different audiences were evident in the responses to the plays' comic elements, particularly gay or Jewish inside jokes, to which clearly distinct sections of the audience laughed at points throughout the play.

Together both plays weave complex themes and symbols in a critique of America's social, economic, and political order, our pervasive religious discourse, millenarian utopianism, and notions of community and family, specifically skewering policies of the Reagan-Bush administrations of the 1980s. Critic John Lahr asserted that *Perestroika's* central issue was the question "Where do love and justice meet?" Tony Kushner himself defined the play's two central questions as the question of forgiveness ("Do you cry for Roy Cohn?") and the question of community and collectivity ("How do you define community?"). Kushner attempted to bring some resolution to these issues in *Perestroika's* problematic final scene, which recapitulates the concerns of both parts of *Angels in America.*[10]

The last scene of the second play is set in Central Park at the Bethesda Fountain, a representation of the biblical Angel of Bethesda, featured in the Gospel of John as a place of healing in Jerusalem. New York's Bethesda Fountain is a memorial to the Union naval dead of the Civil War, America's most thematically apocalyptic conflict. The action of the play includes reconciliation and separation. Kushner wrote a play in two parts in which the monumental evil of Roy Cohn against his own kind—other Jews and other gays—has been forgiven when Louis and the ghost of Ethel Rosenberg pray *Kaddish* over his body in the hospital. Harper has left her husband Joe, who has ended his relationship with Louis. Although Louis has been restored to friendship with Prior, Prior has refused his return as a lover. Thus the play underscores that there are limits to forgiveness and community. Furthermore, in this final scene Prior's best friend Belize negotiates an ambivalent peace with Louis. Hannah Pitt, the Mormon mother who sold everything she owned to come to New York in order to help her stricken son and daughter-in-law, completes this tableau.

A discussion among Belize, Louis, and Hannah on revolution and change is interrupted by Prior's "freezing" the action in order to offer the audience a commentary on their conversation, and at the end, a benediction:

> I'm almost done. . . . This disease will be the end of many of us, but not nearly all, and the dead will be commemorated and will struggle on with the living, and we are not going away. We won't die secret deaths anymore. The world only spins forward. We will be citizens. The time has come. Bye now. You are fabulous creatures, each and every one. And I bless you: *More Life*. The Great Work Begins.

This blessing echoes the last lines of the first play, *Millennium Approaches*, after the angel has broken through the ceiling of Prior's apartment with the announcement:

> Greetings, Prophet;
> The Great Work begins:
> The Messenger has arrived.

The term "great work" was used by alchemists to signify the process of transmuting baser metals into the more perfect gold by means of the "philosopher's stone." In this respect the plays' alchemical trope betrays its influences from Renaissance Neoplatonism as well as Kabbalah mysticism. Later in the twentieth century, psychoanalyst Carl Jung would employ figurative alchemy to discuss the human psyche, particularly in the notion of individuation, the coming-into-being of the Self or the development of human consciousness. Jung postulated that, although alchemists were doing precious little science, they were unconsciously projecting their efforts at self-development. The alchemical ritual was a symbolic process of separation and union, culminating in the *conjunctio* or alchemical marriage of opposites, "allegorized as the mating, fusion, death, and resurrection of . . . the alchemical King and Queen. In a complex, Christian-hermetic symbology, these opposed principles were described in terms of a host of dyadic pairings: light and dark, good and evil, male and female. . . . The outcome of their resolution was the androgynous Adam, the manifestation of divine immortality."[11] Likewise, the play's title, *Perestroika*, the Russian word for "restructuring," a term made familiar in the West by Mikhail Gorbachev's attempts in the 1980s to reform the economy of the Soviet Union, might also be translated by the alchemical term: *transmutation*.

Transmutation is central to Kushner's social homo-utopianism. In the "Afterword" to *Perestroika*, Kushner acknowledged his debt to the writings of Walter Benjamin, whose ideas the playwright discovered through a friend and soulmate, Kimberly T. Flynn. Benjamin's importance for Kushner "rests primarily in his introduction in the 'scientific' disciplines of Marx and Freud a Kabbalist-inflected mysticism and a dark, apocalyptic spirituality" (154), a familiarity with Jewish mysticism that likely can be traced to Benjamin's lifelong friendship with Gershom Scholem, the great twentieth-century scholar of Kabbalah. For example, in "Theses on the Philosophy of History," Benjamin asserted that "the past strives to turn toward that sun which is rising in the sky of history. A historical materialist must be aware of this most inconspicuous of all transformations." Furthermore, "crude and material things" are transmuted into the foundation "without which no refined and spiritual things could exist," while "spiritual things" show themselves "as courage, humor, cunning, and fortitude."[12] Transformation can be viewed as catastrophe or progress, or both, depending on the subject's perspective. Kushner's angel, for instance, is descended from Benjamin's "angel of history" in the ninth thesis, a reflection on Paul Klee's painting "Angelus Novus":

> [H]e is about to move away from something he is fixedly contemplating. His eyes are staring, his mouth is open, his wings are spread. . . . His face is turned toward the past. Where we perceive a chain of events, he sees one single catastrophe which keeps piling wreckage upon wreckage and hurls it in front of his feet. The angel would like to stay, awaken the dead, and make whole what has been smashed. But a storm is blowing from Paradise; it has got caught in his wings with such violence that the angel can no longer close them. This storm irresistibly propels him into the future to which his back is turned, while the pile of debris before him grows skyward. The storm is what we call progress.[13]

Whether one understands Benjamin's angel as a witness to history or the emblem of the historical materialist, the effect in Robert Alter's reading of Benjamin is "a focus on the iconography of tradition [that] serves the purpose of defining more sharply the disasters of secular modernity—the erosion of experience, the decay of wisdom, the loss of redemptive vision, and now, in 1940, the universal reign of mass murder. The angel here is not annunciating angelman but witnessing man, allegorically endowed with the terrible power of seeing things utterly devoid of illusion."[14] Thematically, Kushner's plays ask (but are ambiguous and ambivalent in answering) whether or not a society can be transmuted so that mercy and justice are conjoined.

The most clearly marked transformation of *Angels in America* is Prior's from grief over his AIDS diagnosis and Louis's abandonment of him to wrestling with the angel and demanding "more life." In Act V Scene 5 of *Perestroika*, Prior is permitted to climb the ladder to heaven where he meets with the Continental Principalities, demanding that they take back the Tome of Immobility, the prophecy of stasis that Prior has been asked to proclaim. As he explains to the angelic council:

> We can't just stop. We're not rocks—progress, migration, motion is . . . modernity. It's *animate*, it's what living things do. We desire. Even if all we desire is stillness, it's still desire *for*. Even if we go faster than we should. We can't *wait*.

Similarly, Harper recognizes that she is better off without Joe; Louis, that he has failed Prior, but not failed to love him; Hannah, that opening her heart in compassion is a way more loyal to her faith than strict observance in Salt Lake City, the "right home of the saints." The result in the final tableau is a reconfiguration of the family—an ironic counterpoint to conservatives' atomizing rhetoric in the 1980s and 90s about (nuclear, heterosexual) "family values."

These transmutations are constructions of naive realism, the mimetic plane of "character analysis," and it is likely that *Angels in America* achieved its box office success precisely because of Kushner's strong writing of human particularities and idiosyncrasies in order to represent "character development." However, at the semiosic plane there are more subtle, but for my purposes, more significant, forms of transmutation, a semiotic alchemy if you will.[15] Semioticians have spoken of "transmutation" and "transformation" in a variety of contexts. For example, in discussing the untranslatability of nonlinguistic signs (like music and color) into linguistic signs, Thomas A. Sebeok argued against the possibility of such *intersemiotic transmutation* while Emile Benveniste argued in defense of such translation, a transmutation at least as problematic as the alchemist's. In a more widely accepted formation, Winfried Nöth described language-as-code as a "system of transformation" in which signs in one system replace those in another. Of interest in the present instance, is the notion advanced by the Prague Structuralists that theatrical performance is a site of *semiotic transformation*. Elements that are simply practical in life and would seem only to serve on the mimetic plane (performers, properties, costumes) also signify on the semiosic plane. Performance's roots in ritual are symbolic transformations of lived experience. In addition, in their formulation of a social semiotics, Robert Hodge and Gunther Kress have spent considerable energy articulating a materialist theory of semiotic transformations attempting to "exhume," not gold plates like Joseph Smith or a sacred book in an old suitcase like Prior Walter in *Angels in America*, but the "buried" texts hidden in a cultural product.[16]

Such semiotic transformations are as devilish, if you will pardon the pun, as an alchemist's: they are not material transformations and we can only know them by their effects. Of course, I am troping in the way that Carl Jung or Harold Bloom did in claiming alchemy or Kabbalah, respectively, as structures for their own theories of individuation or the anxiety of influence. What I want to suggest is that while Kushner's *Angels in America* toys thematically with hermetic transformation, he is actually performing transmutation in respect to "symbolic capital," Pierre Bourdieu's term for "accumulated prestige or honour."[17] The plays' effects, at least in terms of print discourse, were remarkable in both number and consensus: New York tabloid and newspaper reviews, newspaper and magazine feature articles, numerous New York theater awards, and a Pulitzer Prize anointed the plays. The long runs that they enjoyed on Broadway, the frequency of regional productions, and an HBO television version directed by Mike Nichols attest to their popular appeal. *Angels in America* produced this response precisely because of the transformative work that Kushner performed on explicitly apocalyptic tropes: prophetic vocation, demonization, and paradisal bliss.

In the stereotypical prophet narratives of the Judeo-Christian tradition, God singles out a worthy man, who may or may not at first accept the call (Jonah, for example, flees from his prophetic calling), but who eventually accepts and fulfills the mission (often, like Jeremiah, lamenting it). If the prophet has any other weakness or sins, these are mitigated by the call. The angelic visitation is a signifier of the authenticity and status of both the calling and the prophet. American angels usually follow this scenario, as in the case of Joseph Smith's believing himself to be called to summon the Saints of the Latter Day. However, angels in American popular culture are likely to perform more personal or individualized missions, consistent with Harold Bloom's characterization of American religion: "The essence of the American is the belief that God loves her or him, a conviction shared by nearly nine out of ten of us, according to a Gallup poll. To live in a country where the vast majority so enjoys God's affection is deeply moving, and perhaps an entire society can sustain being the object of so sublime a regard, which after all was granted only to King David in the whole of the Hebrew Bible."[18] I have in mind the popular belief in "guardian angels" typified in a popular sentimental film, *It's a Wonderful Life*, among other films made before the midcentury, and the *Touched by an Angel* television program popular at the turn of the current century.

Kushner transformed this conventional prophetic/angelic narrative in several ways. First, the prophet, Prior Walter, is doubly stigmatized in the American dominant culture: a gay man with AIDS. The actor playing him in New York and California productions, Stephen Spinella, is extraordinarily slender, with an almost emaciated physique that on the mimetic plane signifies the AIDS wasting syndrome, thus underscoring this impression. Prior, in fact, acknowledges himself to Hannah Pitt as a stereotypical homosexual (*Perestroika* IV iv). Following a conventional biblical pattern, Prior resists the call to prophecy. But instead of eventually repenting, Prior ultimately rejects both the vocation and the message. He returns the sacred text, the Tome of Immobility, to the angels in heaven, admonishing them to accept the inevitability of human agency and change. Kushner invested Prior, and by extension gay men with AIDS like him, with substantial symbolic capital, transmuting him from pariah (or victim) to hero.

Second, although Kushner employed the historical figure of Roy Cohn (described by Louis as "the polestar of human evil . . . the worst human being who ever lived . . ." [*Perestroika* IV ii]), he ultimately asks us to cry for Cohn. In one of *Perestroika*'s most moving scenes, Belize has asked Louis to come to the hospital room where Cohn has just died. Louis is given two tasks: first, to remove the AZT stash that Roy has collected so that Prior can use the medication; and second, to pray the Kaddish, the Jewish prayer for the dead. Belize explains his reason for asking Louis to offer the prayer: "Louis, I'd even pray for you. He was a terrible person. He died a hard death. So maybe . . . A queen can forgive her vanquished foe. It isn't easy, it doesn't count if it's easy, it's the hardest thing. Forgiveness. Which is maybe where love and justice finally meet. Peace, at least. Isn't that what the Kaddish asks for?" (V iii). Louis protests that he is a secular Jew who wasn't even Bar Mitzvahed, which he demonstrates by mistakenly beginning to pray the Kiddush, the prayer for the Friday Sabbath dinner. The ghost of Ethel Rosenberg, who was with Roy when he died, begins to prompt Louis and together they recite the Kaddish. Any excessive sentimentality in the scene, however, is undercut by Louis and Ethel's concluding utterance, "V'imru omain. You sonofabitch." Although a thoroughgoing leftist, Kushner eschewed the kind of predatorial gloating that constituted Robert Sherrill's article in the *Nation*, which the playwright says "equated Cohn's corrupt political life with his sleazy sex life." Kushner remembered being moved by an anonymous panel in the Names Project quilt that read, "Roy Cohn. Bully. Coward. Victim."[19] In a later scene that was cut from the Broadway production, Cohn is depicted, whether in heaven or hell or purgatory is not clear, speaking to God: "Paternity suit? Abandonment? Family court is my particular metier, I'm an absolute fucking demon with Family Law. . . . Is it a done deal, are we on? Good, then I gotta start by telling you you ain't got a case here, you're guilty as hell, no question, you have nothing to plead but not to worry, darling, I will make something up" (V vii).

Kushner similarly resisted stereotyping Hannah Pitt, who otherwise might have been characterized as a mean-spirited Mormon ideologue. (Her one Salt Lake City friend, Sister Ella Chapter, admits, "Know why I decided to like you? I decided to like you 'cause you're the only unfriendly Mormon I ever met" [*Millennium* II x].) After Hannah has moved to New York City and is working as a volunteer at the Mormon Visitor's Center, she meets Prior who has come to the center in search of information on angels. When he collapses with a fever and delirium, she takes him to St. Vincent's hospital. When he regains consciousness, Prior tells Hannah:

PRIOR: I saw an angel. That's insane. . . . She seemed so real. What's happened to me?

HANNAH: You had a vision.

PRIOR: A vision. Thank you, Maria Ouspenskaya. I'm not so far gone I can be assuaged by pity and lies.

HANNAH: I don't have pity. It's just not something I have. One hundred and seventy years ago, which is recent, an angel of God appeared to Joseph Smith in upstate New York, not far from here. People have visions.

PRIOR: But that's preposterous, that's . . .

HANNAH: It's not polite to call other people's beliefs preposterous. He had great need of understanding. Our Prophet. His desire made prayer. His prayer made an angel. The angel was real. I believe that.

PRIOR: I don't. And I'm sorry but it's repellant to me. So much of what you believe.

HANNAH: What do I believe?

PRIOR: I'm a homosexual. With AIDS. I can just imagine what you . . .

HANNAH: No you can't. Imagine. The things in my head. You don't make assumptions about me, mister; I won't make them about you. (IV vi)

A few lines later, after she has told Prior that her son Joe is homosexual, Hannah describes her rage, which she says was not so much about his homosexuality:

HANNAH: But that wasn't it. Homosexuality. It just seems . . . ungainly. Two men together. It isn't an appetizing notion but then, for me, men in *any* configuration . . . well they're so lumpish and stupid. And stupidity gets me cross.

PRIOR: I wish you would be more true to your demographic profile. Life is confusing enough. (IV vi)

As with Kushner's depiction of Roy Cohn, the playwright resisted a facile stereotyping or demonizing of the character, or more particularly in Hannah's case, with her spirituality.

Conversely, because Kushner permitted Louis to be self-absorbed and to abandon Prior, the playwright resisted the sentimentalization of an "AIDS-hero." Instead, although Louis is shown to be devoted to the *idea* of courage and generosity, he falls short of performing courageously or generously, while the Mormon mother of the man who has been Louis's lover extends herself (albeit reluctantly at first) in caring for Prior. Although the characters' naive realism engages the interests of the mainstream audience, the semiosic plane is as significant as the mimetic, especially in regard to signifying difference. By the final tableau, Prior has absorbed and transformed a double stigmatization: the difference of sexuality and the difference of disease. Belize (Norman Arriaga) has absorbed the signs of racial difference: he is not only "black" but also Puerto Rican (Native Caribbean) and colonized (his drag name is also that of a former British colony in Central America). Louis has absorbed the religious and ethnic difference of his Jewishness. Finally, Hannah absorbs the difference of female gender and her Mormon faith. Taken together in the tableau they transform the definition of "family," again not only mimetically representing the kinds of affiliations that gay and lesbian people often produce but also semiosically representing affiliation in difference. These transformations produce in the plays a tremendous moral authority. Kushner takes the moral high road and transmutes the representations of religious symbols from the Judeo-Christian apocalyptic and prophetic conventions, while resisting their ideological rip tides of demonization or of sexual anxiety.

Kushner is a post-Marxian critic. ("[H]is religion is dialectical materialism" according to Don Shewey, though he apparently does not conceive that critique to exclude at least figurative language of spirit.)[20] He proposed what he called, in response to gay assimilationist critics like Andrew Sullivan and Bruce Bawer, "A Socialism of the Skin" that attempts to be simultaneously erotic and pragmatic: "Socialism, as an alternative to individualism politically and capitalism economically, must surely have as its ultimate objective the restitution of the joy of living we may have lost when we first picked up a tool. Towards what other objective is it worthy to strive? . . . Honoring the true desire of the skin, and the connection between the skin and heart and mind and soul, is what homosexual liberation is about."[21] *Angels in America* laments disconnection, whether configured between spouses, lovers, friends, or God with humans. As Kushner offered in a prayer he delivered at New York's Cathedral of St. John the Divine at the National Day of Prayer for AIDS in 1994:

When I was ten an uncle told me you didn't exist. . . . And since his well-meaning instruction I have not *known* your existence, as some friends of mine do; but you have left bread-crumb traces inside of me. Rapacious birds swoop down and the traces are obscured, but the path is recoverable. It can be discovered again. I almost know you are there. I think you are our home. At present we are homeless, or imagine ourselves to be. Bleeding life in the universe of wounds. Be thou more sheltering. God. Pay more attention.[22]

It is in Kushner's association of sex and the sacred that *Millennium Approaches* and *Perestroika* are both wonderfully new and wonderfully ancient. First, the plays refuse to interpret sexuality, desire, or sexual behavior within a binary opposition, conceding that sex has many meanings, sometimes many conflicting meanings in the same sexual act. As he points out in the essay "Fick Oder Kaputt!":

Sex has brought me joy. My people, my community defined by desire. The sweet Joy of Belonging. These are the honeyed leavings of my longings. Sex can be anaesthetic and awakening, abject and exalted, retaliatory and kind, dismal, angelic and pathetic, and all at the same time sometimes—sort of like the twenty hours of the *Ring Cycle* compressed into a few minutes thrashing on a bed.[23]

The plays are also direct in their sexual depictions, as when a guilt-ridden Louis cruises the Ramble of Central Park where he is fucked by a man in leather (*Millennium* II iv) or in *Perestroika* when he and Joe spend their desperate hermetic month together making love in Louis's apartment.

The most important representation of sacred eros occurs in scenes where Prior receives an angelic visitation, which are accompanied inexplicably by his erection and ejaculation. When it first happens to the prophet, he believes that he has only experienced a fever-induced hallucination and wet dream. When the Angel of America appears, s/he (for s/he has eight vaginas and is "REGINA VAGINA! Hermaphroditically Equipped as well with a Bouquet of Phalli . . .") explains the orgasm:

You are Mere Flesh. I I I I am Utter Flesh,
Density of Desire, the Gravity of Skin:
What makes the Engine of Creation Run?
Not Physics But Ecstatics Makes the Engine Run . . .
The Pulse, the Pull, the Throb, the Ooze . . .
Priapsis, Dilation, Engorgement, Flow:
The Universe Aflame with Angelic Ejaculate . . . (*Perestroika* II ii)

While I would imagine that this representation seems blasphemous to some Christians, whose God, angels, and usually saints are scrupulously chaste, it falls squarely within the hermetic traditions of gnosticism, Neoplatonism, Kabbalah, and Mormonism. Some Jewish mysticisms, for example, view marital sexuality as central to salvation, not simply because it sacramentally represents divine fecundity, but because marital intercourse is itself an agent in restoring (*tikkun*) God's female Shekinah from exile and returning her to God's male Yahweh. Human sex, in other words, will bring God together again in a sacred *conjunctio*. Nor is sacred eros a religious antique or esoterica. In his extensive and ongoing sociological study of modern religious consciousness among heterosexuals, Andrew M. Greeley has concluded that, "[a] young adult's religious imagination is most likely to be gracious when he or she is married to a gracious and sexually fulfilling spouse. The combination of sexual fulfillment and a gracious [faith] story told by a spouse is especially powerful for women."[24]

GAY MEN AND SACRED EROS

Gay men did not invent the trope associating eroticism and the sacred, but it has become an important figure affirming sexuality during the AIDS epidemic. For many gay men, post-Stonewall eroticism had absorbed a host of meanings that were central to our individual and communal identities. The prospect that our sexuality might be dangerous did more than threaten to eliminate a source of pleasure; it disturbed the universe we had composed. In Robert Chesley's 1986 play, *Jerker*, two men in San Francisco bond through telephone sex. Though they never meet in the flesh, their relationship develops moments of extraordinary intimacy. The older man, Bert, recalling men's relationships during the 1970s remarks, "But, you know, everyone's putting it down nowadays. . . . 'The party's over! The party's over!' . . . Well, fuck it all, *no! That wasn't just a party*! It was more: a *lot* more, at least to some of us, and it was *connected* to other parts of our lives, *deep* parts, *deep* connections." For Fuzzy and Will in Craig Lucas' 1990 film *Longtime Companion*, set in New York City, sex is eschatological; Fuzzy asks, "What do you think happens when we die?" to which Will replies, "We get to have sex again. I hope." The final scene of the film is a proleptic fantasy of a reunion of those who have died with those who survive.[25] Friends assembled for a funeral in Andrew Holleran's "Friends at Evening" reminisce about the pre-AIDS New York. For one of the men, Ned, the baths were, "A family. A home. A men's club. A place of refuge" where sexual connection was the "whole point, as it were. The central symbol. The Eucharist. What everyone, on some level, was looking for, what everyone would not pause in their search until they found." In a militant reflection on his own living in New York with AIDS, French writer Emmanuel Dreuilhe wrote of himself as one in exile from the homosexual erotic homeland and lamented: "This affirmation of life and shared values is strangely absent from the world of people with AIDS. . . . What we need are art forms that might symbolize our sacred Union, allowing us to identify with our struggle."[26]

The struggle for many gay men in New York and elsewhere in the early 1980s was to make sense of a disease syndrome that was killing their peers in epidemic numbers when they were in the physical and professional prime of their lives. For some this produced a searching examination of their past and reflection on their future, particularly in terms of their own mortality. A variety of Western, Eastern, and alternative religious or spiritual traditions offered many men signs by which to recode the body in its pleasures and pains, or its supplements and losses. Making sense of, or finding meaning in physical devastation became urgent. As a result during the AIDS epidemic, gay men have produced substantial reflections on spirituality and attempted to construct a genealogy of a gay or queer spiritual tradition, many within conventional Western religions and some among Eastern, indigenous, or postmodern spiritualities.

For many AIDS-affected gay men in New York, versions of Western religions or spirituality were the most accessible systems for making sense of life, disease, and death. Their assimilationist agenda produced gay and lesbian communities committed to taking back their own religious traditions on their own terms, resulting in the formation of groups like Dignity for Roman Catholics, Integrity for Episcopalians, the Protestant Fellowship of Metropolitan Community Churches, and other church and synagogue organizations. Probably the most conspicuous of these struggles in church politics has been that in the Roman Catholic Church, which in New York is a lightning rod for a variety of issues. Judaism has been less visibly represented until recently, perhaps because of American Judaism's division into Orthodox, Conservative, and Reformed communities and the decentralized nature of Jewish theological reflection. Nonetheless, as with Kushner, Jewish spirituality also informs the writing of Douglas Sadownick, not only in the novel considered here but also in a later non-fiction book, *Sex Between Men: An Intimate History of the Sex Lives of Gay Men Postwar to Present*, a reappraisal of gay male spirituality.[27] If Kushner's Angel is luminous, Sadownick's is a darkness visible, a fictional representation of the Jungian shadow.

ANGELS IN BLACK LEATHER: DOUGLAS SADOWNICK'S *SACRED LIPS OF THE BRONX*

In the novel *Sacred Lips of the Bronx*,[28] New York-born writer Douglas Sadownick explored autobiographical material in parallel narratives: the adult Michael ("Mikey") Kaplan, a journalist living in Los Angeles, undergoes several limit-experiences while his relationship with performance artist and AIDS activist Robert seems to unravel (Sadownick had been in a relationship with AIDS activist and performance artist Tim Miller for over a decade); and the adolescent Mikey takes as his lover a Puerto Rican-born Hector, a relationship that reaches into the future as Mikey's search for a soulmate. The novel examines the light and shadow aspects of the self, including the reconciliation of opposites that figures in the alchemical process: pain and pleasure, control and surrender, debasement and affirmation, desire and fulfillment. It also participates in the American apocalyptic mythology that situates Paradise to the West of wherever you happen to be, which has had an appeal to Utah Mormons and California New-Age believers alike.[29]

In the novel, while escorting his grandmother, Frieda, to her synagogue, Mikey meets Hector playing basketball with friends. By engaging in contests of symbolic slapping and insulting each other before they become lovers, the two adolescents gradually break down the barrier between Western men and permit their own homosexual desires. After the death of Mikey's grandmother, their relationship grows in intensity until Hector's father discovers that his son is gay. Hector decides to leave New York and wants Mikey to join him in a journey to New Mexico; but at the last moment, Mickey lets Hector leave on the train without him and never sees him again.

As an adult who has made the exodus from the East Coast to the West, Mikey eventually finds himself in a relationship that is deteriorating (his lover, Robert, is having an affair with another AIDS activist) while his own frozen emotional life signals to him that he is heading for a crisis. At the urging of a friend, an African American named John

Drummond (but who is also known as Tahar), Mikey goes to see a Jungian analyst, Myron Smith. Mikey undertakes a journey in the self under the guidance of both Smith in analysis and Tahar, who is an S&M master. With both men, Mikey confronts his own shadow depths and eventually is able to return to New York to visit his and Hector's old neighborhoods and to see his older brother, from whom he has been estranged. Although Mikey and Robert stop living together, they meet at the end of the novel for a meal and a moment of affection and conversation.

Mikey's grandmother Frieda serves as a guiding spirit or guardian over her grandson. After her death, the novel is punctuated by her "visitations" both in his adolescence in New York and in his adulthood in Los Angeles. Toward the end of the novel, Frieda "shows" Mikey his alternative futures, which leaves him better able to accept the past and its production of the present, thus opening the way for the real work of psychotherapy to begin. Since Mikey's assimilationist parents have repudiated Jewish religious practice, Frieda instructs the young man in the lexicon of the spirit:

> Frieda saw the reality behind those lustful images [of Mikey's anonymous sexual encounters before meeting Hector]. To her, the thunder in my skull was the same thunder she saw in her own, . . . But the aching roar was *not* to be found in the closet. Ever look in a porn magazine to find the man or woman of your dreams, only to find out that he or she isn't to be found in a single shot, but rather in the twinge you have in your heart once you close the periodical? Frieda wanted to show me the spirit of her Creator; but this God is invisible. So look instead to the artifacts of your experience; maybe there you will find, if not the world soul, then your own. (262)

Sadownick views his own interest in Judaism as "sublimated homosexuality," suggesting that "religion and homosexuality are soul expressions. They come from a similar place—a transcendent function, a call in the heart."[30] The beloved is a signifier of a desire that predates lovers, parents, and grandparents. In Frieda's last visitation of Mikey, her face changes:

> Into that of Hector? Or rather the memory I had of Hector in his most idealized fashion? My breath swelled into a climax of feeling and longing—a homosexual Beatrice, no? The face smiled benignly, though. The face spoke silent truths: It belonged to both Hector and Frieda— and to neither. . . . This was, then, the soul? . . . The Angel of Death

was also the Angel of Life—wed together in the soul, and by the memories of Frieda and Hector? (288)

Sadownick's tentative assertions are hypotheses, questions posed in twilight rather than bold confessions of faith.

Characterized as "[e]qual parts suffering and bliss," Hector's lips are the sacred lips of the Bronx (233), simultaneously the lips of speech, kissing, licking, and sucking, all of which teach and initiate Mikey into basketball and sexuality:

> He covered my mouth and shook his head. I understood. Hector was not a literal person. Hector would teach me much about words and intentions and actions, which is that they were not the same. Words were both places and names, things that made the heart feel as if it were the dick. Hector would not fuck me that day. Yet he would open up places, like a window opens up places. (119)

Hector is both lover and guide in the education of Mikey's embodied spirit:

> It was this essential education—that we were the same apart from the differences in skin color, language and life's expectations—that was the real interstitial tissue that made up the dream of our future. It was an illusion. But being with Hector taught me that love, which is *not* an illusion, cannot exist without the bad breath and bad jokes and bad faith that come when you get into another person. When that person leaves, he takes his bad things with him. And in his place is an emptiness so huge that your soul cries out for its demons like you wouldn't believe. (231)

Hector also represents the lost twin of Aristophanes' myth in Plato's *Symposium* or gay psychotherapist Mitch Walker's post-Jungian "double," which is neither the Shadow of the Self nor the anima/us, but "a soulmate of intense warmth and closeness" which "embodies the *spirit* of love between those of the same sex . . . [a]nd . . . the supportive ground of the ego."[31] As the Jungian Robert Hopcke employs the notion, the double "serves as the basis for a man's relationship to the masculine in himself and in others. . . . Moreover, both [the double and the anima] function as soul guides for men and lead men into a deeper level of experience of their selves and of the unconscious . . ."[32] Sadownick's obliquely Jungian *Sex Between Men: An Intimate History of the Sex Lives of Gay Men Postwar to Present* adverts in several places to the double. This book offers resistance to the prevailing academic model of sexuality, social constructionism, while overthrowing Freudian "semiotics" and replacing it with Jungian symbolism. Thus instead of "symptoms" signifying "pathologies" Sadownick proposed "symbols" endowed with inexhaustible intelligibility. Sadownick did so in order to caution against a gay man's literalizing his love objects: Analytical depth psychology "offers a way for a gay man to honor his feelings for a lover— or a sex object—in such a way that each encounter creates consciousness, creates an ever-deepening meaningfulness around the riches of symbolic life, even if the encounter hurts."[33]

Through sadomasochistic "scenes," the black AIDS activist John Drummond (Tahar) offers Mikey an opportunity for deepened consciousness and guides him through his own griefs that have resulted from the loss of Hector, the loss of Robert's fidelity, and the loss of friends to AIDS. In much the same way as Hector was ethnically "other," Tahar's blackness signifies his Jungian "shadow" status to Mikey, who as a journalist and a Jew is more at home with the Apollonian configurations of his emotional and erotic life. After soaking Mikey in a hot bath, Tahar binds him to a cross in the sound-proofed "playroom" of his home while instructing his initiate:

> "Now listen up, whiteboy. This is not about pain for pain's sake. If something hurts you too much, just say stop, okay? And we'll stop. But also see how far you can go, okay? Let yourself relax into it; see it all as medicine. So look, you have two jobs. One: breathe. Deep breaths in, nice soft ones out. Two: scream. . . . But think of your screams as, well, you know, sacred. I mean, don't shit them out, but see if you can make them come from your heart, not your throat, if you know what I mean." (98)

For Tahar, this scene does not signify hedonistic pleasure in pain for its own sake but pain as a shamanistic healing ritual, about a man's trusting and letting go with another man. Adopting a vaguely Hebraic "drag name," Tahar is a black leather angel. Having blocked his own grief, Mikey finds that the S&M sessions with Tahar permit him to wail and require him to reestablish trust with himself and with another. This dynamic in their fictional relationship is consistent with Thomas Moore's observation in *Dark Eros: The Imagination of Sadism* that:

> Most of us know that sex offers exuberant sensations of vitality, but we also know that it asks for a continuous stretching of the structures of

life and our understanding. We might like to have both the feeling of vibrancy and familiar structures and interpretations, but ultimately these reveal themselves to be in contradiction. Sade's libertines engage in regular rituals of erotic exploration intent upon discovering ever new ways of satisfying the need for pleasure. Perhaps these rituals say something about the soul's work, its liturgy, as an endless exploration of the demands of desire. Opening up to those desires is the only route to the sense of being fully alive that most of us crave.[34]

The S&M scenes produce an altered state of consciousness for Mikey equivalent to the weeping rapture of a Pentecostal believer, whereby the physical pain induces him to express the emotional pain. After another session with his therapist and S&M scene with Drummond, Mikey relates that "Tahar's deep laughter begins to ease my fears that Myron is Satan and Tahar is his Prince of Darkness minion. I trust Tahar—or, more to the point, I trust his body. . . . Now, Myron seems more well-meaning, if impatient. 'Impatient with all the gay men dying before they know who they are,' Tahar adds" (182–3).

Myron Smith's therapy is the analytical version of Tahar's S&M scenes. He is firm and unrelenting in requiring that Mikey face his own shadow-self. When at a crucial point in the therapy Mikey resists and angrily walks out of the session, Myron roars at his client:

> "No, you're nuts. . . . Or, rather, you're not nuts enough. You're hollow in your nuttiness, wrapped around by it, but not embracing it, led around like a dog who doesn't know his own master. You dare to use the Self's name in vain. When was the last time you talked to God, you phony. You come in here and talk about your lover and your dog, and then you use the Self's name as a curse. If you leave here, you'll be cursed to walk the earth like a leper, a leper of feelings, a vampire, a vampire feeding off other men, with no soul of your own, chasing the secret of your life like a dog chases his own tail." (180)

Mikey reacts to this attack by knocking over and shattering a Greek vase in the therapist's waiting room, emptying its ironic contents: miniature dog bones, one of which Myron gives to Mikey signifying his successful negotiation of another stage in the therapy. Later when Mikey has resisted the allure of Frieda's ghostly offer of alternative futures and after the chance meeting with a stranger, Luis, who bears an uncanny resemblance to Hector, Myron can announce, "Now . . . we can get to work"

(289). The reader wants Mikey's reunion with the lost twin, or at least perhaps a moment's satisfaction of ancient hungers with Luis, but Myron (and Sadownick) reminds us that the construction of the Self (Jung's "individuation") is work.

Individuation has social implications that Sadownick placed in the center of his later project, *Sex Between Men*, which proposed to be not only an analytical psychosexual history of gay men in the second half of the twentieth century but also a program for gay male community into the twenty-first century. Just as AIDS, like a radioactive dye, has penetrated and revealed the fault lines of individual relationships in *Sacred Lips of the Bronx*, so the health crisis exposed similar fissures in larger collectives of gay men in North America. While Sadownick acknowledged the extent of many gay men's spiritual introspection with the beginning of the crisis, the second post-AIDS crisis of prevention, ably documented more recently by Walt Odets and others,[35] has argued compellingly that gay men may have produced short-term management of a crisis, but that the longer term issues remain unresolved. Epidemiological statistics show an increase in HIV infection among older and younger gay men, the first who ought to know better but for whom years of epidemic anxiety have taken their toll. Many gay men are still highly susceptible to the commodification of sexuality, and impossible physical ideals leave older gay men (35 and above!) feeling as though they have little to live for if they can no longer attract a partner. This consumerist ideology renders many men vulnerable to unsafe sex practices (as well as to other risky behaviors). The resulting alienation, Sadownick pointed out, "can offer either the greatest of possible opportunities or the most devastating of catastrophes" (229). In addition, he noted that while there have been "scattered attempts to create indigenous community spaces that had as their main purpose an effort to connect Eros with Culture" (229), these (like the utopian politics of ACT UP and Queer Nation) have been short-lived.

Sadownick suggested that erotic extroversion needs to be balanced with introversion. Many gay men had become so self-identified with genital sexuality that it constituted their persona, which is "another way of saying 'our social self,' a collective way of adapting to the world" (237). Part of the mythology of "gay" has been its typically American insistence on the brightly positive or optimistic registers of human experience, "[b]ut once the equation is made between gay = happy, then what kind of space is left for someone experiencing and working with unhappiness or existential pain[?]" (239). More to the point, the search for bonding which pervades even gay erotica, in Sadownick's revised Jungianism, employs a complex emotional alchemy:

> [T]he man provoking the crush is no mere man but also a screen for the projection of soul, with all the weight and potential that loaded word implies. We are throwing onto our lovers the best and worst part of the Self when we fall for them. Romantic love is nothing but projection, but a fabulous one. To become more and more aware of this psychic phenomenon is not to stymie love, but rather to become a more artful player in the steamy cycles of projection and recollection, falling in love as well as owning that feeling as one's own and seeing how that could take one into new dimensions of being. (241).

This introversion, however, entails a degree of self-examination and ego-strength that would not seem to be hallmarks of American culture and social life.

Sadownick's faith in analytical depth psychology is also tinged with American millennialist hopes in the kingdom of the West. In *Sex Between Men* he collected "West Coast gay-centered thinkers" like Harry Hay, Mitch Walker, Mark Thompson, Don Kilhefer, Robert Hopcke, and Joseph Kramer, and he claimed that "[w]hat separates this new spiritual outlook from gays going to their Jewish and Hindu temples or Christian and crystal churches is that the power of gay psyche as these thinkers see it is rooted specifically in gayness and the latent divinity said to reside there; it needn't borrow from institutions with a history of persecuting gays" (238–39). This statement represents a remarkably ingenuous faith in a "prelapsarian" analytical discourse free of the messy complications of ideology or history. Furthermore, Sadownick believes in the existence of unmediated prediscursive experience. In a footnote in which he criticized Judith Butler's (and academics' generally)[36] " 'materialist' arrogance" Sadownick asserted:

> Of course, the minute one writes down a dream, one changes its representation from "pure" to "written" form. But so what? One could argue that the symbolic *feeling* one has in working with the dream is *pure*, is *essential*, is *experiential*. The nightmare gets the heart beating, it incarnates a certain truth. Butler argues things on the level of "concepts" but what if one brings feeling to bear on thinking? What if the imaginal world, the world of psyche, is more real than the world of

discourse? What if the unconscious originates, causes, and composes? (244 n12)

Even a revised Jungianism is nonetheless implicated in its own discursive history, in the ideological formations that compose that discourse, and which that discourse represents. For example, in reading Jung, analytic practitioners often approach his writings as sacred texts requiring the preservation of a canonical tradition. However, all traditions (*traditio*) are betrayals (*proditio*), both to their patriarchs and to their subjects. What Jungians and some post-Jungians betray specifically is a dedication to gendered binarisms (for example, the *animus* and *anima*) of the kind that have been so problematic to gay and lesbian people in the twentieth century. While insisting that Jung over Freud offers a more liberatory understanding of sexuality and gender, recent post-Jungian feminists acknowledge that "[w]hen Jung's personal associations to feminine qualities and masculine qualities were projected into his analytical psychology, they became static. It is as if the archetypes fell into matter and re-emerged as stereotypes."[37] In this regard, Carol Schreier Rupprecht has mapped four areas where Jung's work inadequately represented women: "the tendency toward dualism; the sanctifying ontology accompanying archetypal images ascribed to the female; confusion of enculturated social roles with actual gender identity; and the tendency to define the female predominantly through her relation to the male"; and she proposed that, "If we are to become feminist archetypal readers of texts and interpreters of dreams, we must leave the animus behind once and for all."[38]

Furthermore, Sadownick's belief in "pure" experience, that is unmediated by discourse, betrays either a narrow understanding of "discourse" or a naive understanding of consciousness, which is always already configured in terms of difference and sameness, the semiotic system that constitutes perception and affect or emotion, as well as language. "Experience" for humans is never prediscursive, but Sadownick needs to imagine its possibility because Jung's version of Neoplatonism posits a world of ideal forms, the archetypes that transcend cultures and are a foundation of Sadownick's utopian faith. This permits him the Romantic idealism that makes *Sacred Lips of the Bronx* so imaginative and *Sex Between Men* so problematic.

Not all post-Jungians have been that naive. In "The Unconscious in a Postmodern Depth Psychology," Paul Kugler explored the deconstructive potentialities in post-Jungianism by examining the central concept of the

unconscious, within structuralist, Lacanian, and poststructuralist readings of the term. By categorizing Jung as a structuralist, Kugler was able
to admit that "the unconscious" is a discursive representation and thus a
signifier of something unknowable, one of many *"temporal and linguistic
by-products* resulting from a representational theory of language. Any
such transcendental *term* is a fiction, heuristically and clinically valuable,
perhaps, but nonetheless fictional." He proposed a hermeneutic strategy
similar to the one that Paul Ricoeur once characterized as a "second
naivete," namely that:

> In therapeutic analysis we still must, on one level, *believe in* our god
> term [e.g., "the unconscious"] and use it *as if* it were the ultimate
> explanatory principle. But on a deeper level, we also know that it is
> not. And it is precisely this deeper level of awareness that prevents our
> psychological ideologies from becoming secular religions and differen-
> tiates professional debates from religious idolatry. For the ultimate ground
> of depth psychology is not a known god term but the ultimately un-
> knowable, the unconscious itself.[39]

Sadownick's desire for a prelapsarian and prelinguistic "experience" is
understandable. However, in literalizing the trope of Eden he runs the
risk of an authoritarian politics in which sovereignty is granted to those
who can persuade an audience of the prelapsarian "purity" of their "experience." These are typical perils of gnosticism and hermeticism, and are
all the more urgent given Jung's concern about totalitarianism.[40] Similarly, Sadownick's characterization of semiotics and Freudianism as sign
systems (pointing to the known) in contrast to Jungian analysis as a
symbol system (pointing to the unknown) is a flawed critique. As David
L. Miller points out in "An Other Jung and An Other . . . ," citing James
Hillman, the symbolic order and the semiotic have exchanged places over
time: "symbolism is the domain of the known (or what the collective
leads us to think we know), which leaves the sign world to be the locus
of the unknown. Signs situate us in dislocations without semantic security, not in the subject or in the object, but in the abject."[41]

Sadownick's utopianism in *Sex Between Men* deserves careful examination, even though I believe it is flawed, because it also has some important things to say about the "inner" life (again, an admittedly troubling
spatial trope) of gay men in the United States in the second AIDS decade
at the end of the second millennium. The imaginative achievement of

Sacred Lips of the Bronx makes Sadownick an authoritative writer. In offering a critique of his later book, I find myself resonating with David Miller's justification for his own deconstruction of Jung:

> What does any of this matter? It is to the end of the continual alchemical process of dynamic unsettling that allows one to see from the perspective of the Other. (Therapists in Jung's day were called "alienists," from *alius* = "other.") It is in order to deconstruct unconsciousness, ideology, and idolatry. Indeed, the other Jung opens to Otherness as a possibility in the time of the death of the ego (the subject), in the time of the death of symbolisms (object-relations), and in the time of the death of other gods as well.[42]

Hope is an act of imagination, and a reconciliation with the Others composed as "opposite" requires imagination. As Peggy Phelan has written, "the hope we fake and perform and the hope we thereby make and have. Hope's power is measured in this faking. Each performance registers how much we want to believe what we know we see is not all we really have, all we really are."[43] Utopias are always doomed from the start because Eden and Progress are both fictions. Still that doesn't stop us from telling stories about both. Sadownick ended *Sacred Lips of the Bronx* with the separated Robert and Mikey holding hands in a restaurant, a moment of *convivium* and *conjunctio*. He did something similar in *Sex Between Men*:

> For too long, moralists have equated wisdom with the renunciation of hot sex. What a scam. The odyssey of gay life over five decades proves at least this much: that a magical thread links one's third eye with one's cock. Yes a man must go out of himself to find the stud he dreams of. . . . And yes, often the search throws the person back into his own unfathomable depths. . . . Whatever the dangers in sex, gay men's innate drive to make love to other men (one or many) corrects, redeems, and intervenes in a world gone mad with man-to-man violence. There may be a greater intelligence in Eros than we can grasp—for now. Desire seizes that man whose soul has been brushed by another man's kiss and, holding him by the collar says: This is your existence—and it is natural, it is positive, it is good, and it is spinning a new way to be. Developing greater and greater mindfulness about this powerful inner call seems likely to become the emergent gay myth for the future. (242)

Sadownick resisted easy bromides about "closure" or even "hope." Conjunction is often a dark, violent mystery and ecstasy is often a divine delirium. He invited his gay male readers to be awake, not narcotized by addiction or compulsion, and to resist pre-packaged assimilationist fantasies.

ASSIMILATION AND UTOPIANISM

For many (indeed, perhaps most) gay and lesbian Americans, Paradise looks like a familiar city neighborhood, suburb, or small town. How does one maintain a dialectic between sameness and difference in American society? Are the terms of that question themselves hopelessly implicated in a reductionist binarism? What are the terms of acceptance (or is it surrender?) into a dominant culture and what room is there for resistance through difference? Both Tony Kushner's *Angels in America* and Douglas Sadownick's *Sacred Lips of the Bronx* wrestle with those questions and to some extent represent "homo-utopias" based on this edgy negotiation between assimilation and marginality. In both the plays and the novel, religious communities, transmuted into ethnic minorities, are presented as paradigms of assimilation. Kushner's Mormons and Jews and Sadownick's Jews are case studies of the losses and gains entailed in the dialectic between assimilation and marginality. Once a despised sect, driven out of the Midwest United States to a desert in Utah, Mormonism now finds its disciples in high-status positions, its wealth established, its votes courted by politicians. Although Jewish communities have existed in North America since the colonial period, massive European immigrations in the nineteenth and twentieth centuries, particularly into urban areas, brought people who were different in terms of class and nationality; these too have assimilated to a remarkable degree. In both cases, Mormons and Jews in North America have often sought assimilation while simultaneously maintaining their own physically separate enclaves. For *Angels in America*, Joe Pitt and Roy Cohn represent the worst excesses of assimilationism, while Hannah Pitt seems to maintain both her Mormon beliefs and a rapport with the morally marginalized. Louis, who is an almost cartoonishly assimilated secular Jew, seems soulless. Prior and Belize are certainly the most significantly marginalized characters. One is a drag enthusiast with AIDS; the other, an Afro-Puerto Rican, yet they both concede to some of the demands of the larger dominant culture. In *Sacred Lips of the Bronx*

Mikey's sympathy with his grandmother's Jewish orthodoxy is a source of embarrassment to his assimilated parents for whom religious practice signifies exclusion from American middle-class culture.

Assimilation is another form of transmutation within cultural alchemy. In *The Angel and the Beehive: The Mormon Struggle with Assimilation*, Armand L. Mauss observes, "In what might be called the 'natural history' of the interaction between radical social movements and their host societies, there seem to be no historical exceptions to the proposition that new movements must either submit to assimilation in important respects or be destroyed." However, he also characterizes the survival of dissident communities as a dialectic between two forces: "the strain toward greater assimilation and respectability, on the one hand, and that toward greater separateness, peculiarity, and militance on the other. Along the continuum between total assimilation and total repression or destruction is a narrow segment on either side of the center; and it is within this narrower range of socially tolerable variation that movements must maintain themselves, pendulumlike, to survive."[44] In addition, Mauss cites historian R. Laurence Moore's contention in *Religious Outsiders and the Making of Americans* which "maintains that 'outsider' status has been almost a cherished possession for new religions in America, validating simultaneously (and ironically) both their unique claims to heavenly sanction and their quintessential Americanness."[45] Mauss points out that while deviant groups (using the term in its sociological sense, not moralizing sense) are agents of change in dominant cultures, it is usually the case that the deviant group must renounce more of its claims to distinction, a pattern he claims for Mormonism which moved from some of its nineteenth-century hermetic beliefs and the practice of polygamy to more mainstream Protestant beliefs and sexual practice. These beliefs and practices changed when Mormon leaders claimed a new prophecy to warrant their adoption. (Americans, after all, can tolerate more theological peculiarity than erotic.) Finally, Mauss notes that from the mid-twentieth-century Mormons have increasingly been characterized as an ethnic group, transmuting "peculiarity" into "ethnicity," a construction that prompts him to draw Mormon/Jewish parallels. This dialectic suggests to me two things: first, the fluidity of "identity" and the constructedness of "ethnicity"; second, the weakness of the binarism "assimilation" and its "opposite," "marginality," or "resistance."

I want to suggest that in the cultural dialectic between assimilation and marginality, gay people's difference is more like Jewish people's difference than it is like black people's difference, while I acknowledge the constructedness of those differences. Although "race" and "ethnicity" are fictions, they are in some respects two distinct fictions. While those fictions are often used to exclude the Other from symbolic and cultural capital, they are probably also employed just as often as a means of inclusion within a collective. Jonathan Rauch has suggested the gay/Jewish analogy that:

> Jews recognize that to many Americans we will always seem different (and we are in some ways, different). We grow up being fed "their" culture in school, in daily life, even in the calendar. It never stops. For a full month of every year, every radio program and shop window reminds you that this is, culturally, a Christian nation (no, not Judeo-Christian). Jews could resent this, but most of us choose not to, because, by way of compensation, we think hard, we work hard, we are cohesive, and we are interesting. We recognize that minorities will always face special burdens of adjustment, but we also understand that with those burdens come rewards of community and spirit and struggle.[46]

While most self-identified American "gay" or "lesbian" people seek the same social and economic goals as other middle-class Americans, we also often identify with our difference, frequently to the point of composing exceptionalist fictions about ourselves (we are more talented, more aesthetic, more interesting than straight people). And while discourse about AIDS has been stigmatizing, the "spectacle of AIDS" (to use Simon Watney's term) has paradoxically also fostered a gay visibility that represents us as courageous, compassionate, and resourceful. Would that those stories could have been told without an epidemic! Thus Utopia is literally "nowhere" and yet we continue to tell utopian stories to keep the alchemy going. In other words, I am arguing for an "alchemy" of assimilation and separatism, culturally and politically, much like that evident in *Angels in America* and *Sacred Lips of the Bronx*.[47]

The cultural politics that I have in mind has been described by Steven Seidman in "Identity and Politics in a 'Postmodern' Gay Culture: Some Historical and Conceptual Notes." In defining "postmodernism" Seidman contends it is a "speaking of multiple, local, intersecting struggles whose aim is less 'the end of domination' or 'human liberation' than the creation of social spaces that encourage the proliferation of pleasures, desires, voices, interests, modes of individuation and democratization."[48]

As such, a postmodern cultural politics has to be suspicious of fictions of monolithic unitary identity and alert to our multiple (and competing if not conflicting) subject positions. Seidman's proposal is explicitly antiapocalyptic:

> I urge a shift away from the preoccupation with self and representations characteristic of identity politics and poststructuralism to an analysis that embeds the self in institutional and cultural practices. I favor a politics of resistance that is guided by a transformative and affirmative social vision. This suggests an oppositional politic that intends institutional and cultural change without, however, being wedded to millennial vision.[49]

Such an approach is by extension also antifoundational:

> I prefer a pragmatic approach to social criticism. Conceptual and political decision making would be debated in terms of concrete advantages and disadvantages; the values guiding such pragmatic calculus would receive their moral warrant from local traditions and social ideals, not foundational appeals. In a pragmatically driven human studies, I imagine critical analyses that address specific conflicts, aim to detail the logics of social power, and do not shy away from spelling out a vision of a better society in terms resonant to policy makers and activists.[50]

It is as an activist that I come to urge Seidman's praxis. For the last twenty years I have joined others in carrying out resistance raids on heteronormativity in a variety of less-than-hospitable fields: the plains of East Central Illinois when I was a graduate student at the University of Illinois, in the priesthood of the Roman Catholic Church, and among the military and evangelical communities of Southern Virginia. Experiences and conversations with other activists suggest to me that pragmatics are a useful way of mediating the competing claims of assimilationism and separatism; likewise, perhaps, the competing claims of queer realism and idealism. As our leaning toward hermetic traditions suggests, we are very much the heirs of Platonic binarism, in ways that often have been played out as conflicts between "body" and "spirit," which are themselves signifiers of longed-for presences. Our object choices—erotic or utopian—signify the gap between, on the one hand, our desires and imaginings, and on the other, our capacities. Homosexual desires find Eden very lonely and so fancy another place that is both lost and yet to come.

HOMO-UTOPIAS

Throughout this chapter I have tried to show AIDS utopianism's relationship to Anglo-American culture and history, particularly in the hermeticism that is characteristic not only of specific religious practices like Mormonism or Jewish mysticism, but also of "American religion" generally as Harold Bloom characterizes it. Nineteenth-century homosocialists like Herman Melville and Charles Warren Stoddard imagined their ideal places with sailors on ships or with indigenous peoples on Pacific islands.[51] Gay Northern Europeans were similarly fascinated with the Mediterranean world as an idealized site of unfettered erotic expression, imaginings that were wedded to Western colonialist discourses and an aesthetic *topos* that may also be akin to literary Arcadian conceits.[52] In an unfinished essay, the late Tom Yingling suggested, "Whitman discovers that homosexual utopia is not a place but a practice; and if homosexual utopia is a strategy of displacement rather than a future site of social perfection, 'Calamus' demonstrates that one of the things that needs to be displaced is 'America,' " a view not dissimilar to Fabian Socialists like Edward Carpenter, the early twentieth-century thinker and writer on homosexual relations. The rural idyll at Milthorpe of Carpenter and his mate George Merrill was recast in the form of the novel *Maurice* after E. M. Forster visited the pair.[53] A homosexual literary tradition imagines Utopias of erotic bliss where desire and loss are transmuted into signifiers of vitality.

Not all AIDS-affected discourse, however, supports utopianism. Gay conservative Bruce Bawer has criticized Tony Kushner's article "Socialism of the Skin" and claimed a consensus: "more and more gay people are impatient with the queer left's abiding fascination with aimless utopianism; we're impatient with models of activism that involve playing at revolution instead of focusing on the serious work of reform . . . rather than a self-indulgent millenarianism full of sound and fury, signifying nothing."[54] Insofar as Bawer calls for a *realpolitik*, his critique might be valuable, but whose *realpolitik*? Socialist writer and activist Scott Tucker replies:

> Let's grant that the utopian impulse *can* be dangerous. And what else is the corporate dream of the New World Order, if not business as usual till the kingdom come? Isn't this also crazed and corrupt? Wilde made the point—in a dandyish manner calculated to irk all puritans—that real democracy and individualism are only possible when leisure, pleasure, and justice are not reserved for the few.[55]

One person's visionary thinking is another's "aimless utopianism." Utopia is not inherently a delusion or false ideology. The dangers of utopianism, however, are akin to those of Christian millennialism: literal and ahistorical readings prevent democratic compromise, endorsement of provisional gains, and acknowledgement of material complexities. Implicit in the texts that I have examined throughout this study is the belief that there are better ways of ordering human relations than the existing dominant order. In particular, they embrace the conjunction of pleasure and responsibility, a concept not terribly foreign to the American foundational (and, given the extent to which its work is unfulfilled, utopian) text that asserts inalienable rights to life, liberty, and the pursuit of happiness.

If heedless hedonism seemed the utopian dream of many gay men in the 1970s, AIDS woke many of us up in the 1980s. Instead, we discovered responsible pleasure, not only because our individual lives depended on it, but also because we came to see our individualism as contingent upon collective solidarity. David Drake and Tim Miller's performance pieces endorsed erotic bliss in the context of AIDS activism. James McCourt's *Time Remaining* mixed memory and desire not in a ritual of camp nostalgia but in the liturgy of survival. Although a scold, Larry Kramer did not repudiate desire or pleasure, and his autobiographical plays demonstrate his willingness to imagine human relations rescued from past calamities. Figures like Sarah Schulman, and groups like ACT UP and Lesbian Avengers demonstrated discipline and solidarity on behalf of the body and its pleasures, producing results that still reverberate in direct action campaigns (such as World Trade Organization protests) and in the expeditious way with which promising medical treatments are now often made available. Third World countries dealing with AIDS today have paid attention to those successes and are using them to advocate for treatment of their citizens. Tony Kushner and Douglas Sadownick urged audiences and readers to imagine human interconnectedness and complexity, to interrogate sanitized utopian fantasies (either those of the free market or of ideological purity), and to risk the provisional compromises and small gains that can lead to new human relations. In what has to be one of the strangest paradoxes of the AIDS crisis, queer people in the United States are now irrevocably at the table (although we may not like everything on the menu and some of our neighbors refuse to pass us the salt). This awkward assimilation into American life can hardly be called a homo-utopia, but utopianism made it possible by making it thinkable.

With the development of combination drug therapies, AIDS in the industrialized world has become a manageable illness, for those who can afford the drugs. This medical breakthrough requires cognitive breakthroughs as well. Shortly after the introduction of "drug cocktails," the local AIDS service organization, on whose community advisory board I have served, referred to me a young man with AIDS (diagnosed when he was in high school) who wanted to apply for admission to the college where I teach. "I've spent the last ten years getting ready to die," he told me. "Now I want to get ready to live." We can at the very least imagine life without AIDS (even if not one without HIV). Whether it is a socially constructed discursive formation or a genetically "hard wired" function of the brain or a spiritual gift (or all three), hope often enables survival while we are waiting for *nowhere* to become *now here*.

Afterword

(In)conclusion

(In memory of Roger)

In July 1981 while attending a month-long summer institute at the University of San Diego, California, I spent a four-day weekend in a city I had never visited, San Francisco. Alone for the weekend, I walked its streets as an energetic tourist intending to compress as many gay sites and tourist sights as possible into the brief visit. Very quickly I found myself in the company of the loneliness that I have tried to evade for decades, which I attempted to remedy by seeking all the usual places where gay men can find each other: an adult book store, a pornographic film theater, several Castro Street bars, and the opera house. However, I returned to San Diego untouched. Although I met and chatted up several men in San Francisco, I went home with no one. I yearned for it and I feared it. Paradoxically, I had locked out of house and home many of my desires, and since I denied them an honorable domesticity, they continued to vandalize me for several more years. To put it more directly, I was terrorized by the briny convulsions of gay male sexuality.

The month before my visit to San Francisco, the *San Francisco Chronicle* reported on "A Pneumonia That Strikes Gay Males."[1]

What does it *mean*, what is the *significance* of this fact, that I have survived the AIDS epidemic and remained HIV negative? During the 1970s and early 80s, I had engaged in some of the sexual behaviors that put one at risk for HIV infection. Even more astonishing, in San Francisco during July 1981, how could I have failed to find a sexual partner under the circumstances: a 28-year-old tourist visiting the gay Mecca of

177

North America at the height of its erotic exuberance? Behind that lurks another question: What is the meaning of asking, "What does it mean?"

The first question is sort of a blank screen on which I can project a variety of my inherited cultural and discursive referents. The Angel of Death passed over me. Or anxiety about sexuality per se and guilt about my homosexual desires produced a reaction formation in which I was policing the unruliness of eros by strictly defining the boundaries of my own body to avoid what I had configured as physical "defilement" and erotic "danger." Or "inheriting" my mother's health neuroses and alert to the medical concerns already circulating among gay men, I was consciously or unconsciously avoiding infection by herpes, hepatitis, or other sexually transmitted diseases. Or by the laws of statistical probability in a complex chaotic universe (and this mechanism is now confirmed by epidemiology), most gay men in the United States simply are not HIV infected, and, therefore, I fell among those in the "lucky" category, which is itself a fictional construction of a universe interested in our concerns. Or I am a "survivor" with a mission to bear witness. Or God saved me for a purpose. Or amazing grace. Or blind chance. Or all of the above. Settling on any one interpretation is reductive; what the AIDS epidemic "means" is greater than the sum of all of them taken together. Or it means nothing. Moreover, its various "meanings" compete and conflict. None of them may be verifiable, but any of them can be meaningful; that is, in Robert Hodge and Gunther Kress's terms, those narratives perform valuable "semiosic work." Thus even to assert that AIDS is "meaningless" is to place the epidemic within a horizon of signification that paradoxically asserts its meaningfulness by denying it.

While any one of these mythologies is perhaps as good or bad as any other, the more beguiling question is the second: What does it mean that I (along with many others) am compelled to compose a meaning for my evasion of infection? From where comes our need for semiosic work? How does it continue to operate in ways that are harmful or helpful?

Earlier in this study I acknowledged the inevitability of signification in the absence of any prelinguistic or unmediated "experience." Paula Treichler has famously called HIV/AIDS an "epidemic of signification," although AIDS is not alone in evoking such a response; perhaps it is just more overtly so. This study has examined not only certain kinds of signification—apocalyptic tropes of exile, prophetic jeremiad, Armageddon, and paradise—but at least indirectly has interrogated the systems and mechanisms of signification themselves and the desires that generate and sustain them. Particularly, I have been concerned with the discursive production of "identities," which are repertoires of signifying practices, performances, rather than essences. In most of the cases considered here, culture workers—including artists, performers, intellectuals, and AIDS educators—have argued less over the fact of human signification than over the specific signifiers employed. For example, Susan Sontag warned against a metaphorical signification of all diseases, including AIDS. Sarah Schulman argued against constructing a soteriological trajectory for AIDS narratives and insisted that there is no redemptive meaning to the epidemic.

Those of us who are "AIDS survivors" (itself a trope) have frequently asked ourselves what "surviving" or being "spared" *means*. Shortly after the onset of the epidemic, in private collectives and in public discourse, gay men began to ask if there was a "message" in the epidemic, a meaning to be construed, or a "lesson" to be learned. Probably the only certain message, meaning, or lesson is that humans cannot live long without construing a message, meaning or lesson, and in the largely Protestant-derived culture of the United States, a typological interpretation of material events is almost compulsory. Discourse, as Hodge and Kress point out, has both semiosic and mimetic planes; that is to say, it both conveys messages and claims representational authority, though often, as in the case of American apocalypticism, the distinction between the two planes seems without a difference. Both message and mimesis make implicit claims for authority, and AIDS discourse in the United States has been a contest among competing and often conflicting ideologies.

Throughout this study I have suggested that there has been a kind of inevitability to apocalyptic tropes, given the pervasiveness of apocalypticism within the hegemonic Protestantism of the United States. At the same time, however, I have cautioned against too neat a distinction between "dominant" and "marginal" discourses, precisely because of the fluidity in our semiotic systems, metonymic of the fluidity of "identity." The complexity of postmodern subject positions makes this binarism impossible to sustain. I have also argued that apocalyptic discourse is determined to polarize binary opposites, which it concocts through a variety of anxiety-producing figures, such as physical penetration and defilement. Whatever necessary fictions "AIDS survivors" inscribe as our Burkean "equipment for living" with loss and fear, we have to be alert to their by-products and contraindications.[2] As Lee Quinby points out in her subtle and careful analysis, *Anti-Apocalypse: Exercises in Genealogical Criticism*:

Apocalypticism in each of its modes fuels discord, breeds anxiety or apathy, and sometimes causes panic. Decision-making suffers when it takes apocalyptic form—whether at the level of individual, everyday personal choices or of local, national, and international government, military, and peace-keeping deliberations. What makes apocalypse so compelling is its promise of future perfection, eternal happiness, and godlike understanding of life, but it is that very will to absolute power and knowledge that produces its compulsions of violence, hatred, and oppression.

Apocalypse often implies genocide. Although the Western world claimed to have witnessed enough of that by the middle of the twentieth century, it remained impassive toward the close of the century as new world orders disposed of the old in Cambodia, Iraq, Bosnia, Rwanda, and elsewhere. Similarly, inured by AIDS apocalypticism as political rhetoric, the West has been unable to fathom its mimetic possibilities in Africa, where populations are HIV infected with an incidence unimagined in North America. As William Haver cautions:

> By the terms of its logic, of course, the thought of the apocalypse can only be a figure in the historical Imaginary because the apocalypse can only be situated in the future, always postponed for existing beings. Which makes the apocalypse that which identifies those who envision the apocalyptic to be, in fact, oracular seers or prophets, witnesses to a future that is the end of the very possibility of futurity. The effects of this apocalyptic Imaginary have been traced often enough: to envision the apocalypse makes us of us [sic], here and now, tragic heroes devoted . . . to that destruction which would be, not only our consolation, but our redemption, our resurrection. But this tragic devotion to the figure of a redemptive apocalypse . . . denies the very possibility of futurity, of praxis, of what is called agency, of anything, indeed, except the valorization of . . . the obliteration of possibility itself . . .

Thus, while apocalyptic discourse is often framed in such a way as to enjoin action, a contrary and entropic desire for inaction frequently renders apocalyptic subjects inert.[3]

At the same time, apocalypticism is appealing for two reasons: first, it makes all cohere, and second, it is inherently narcissistic, which appeals particularly to Americans' insatiable hunger for attention. Apocalypticism is to history what chaos theory is to physics, that is an attempt to provide a unified macro-theory that explains every microphenomenon. Every historical event, no matter how seemingly random or chaotic or minute is explained by the apocalyptic plot as either divinely ordained or demonically instigated. At the same time, apocalyptists believe themselves to be personally engaged in the plot of a cosmic drama, performing a star turn in the eschatological spectacle. Thus the eighteenth-century American preacher and theologian Jonathan Edwards living in a small Massachusetts town and twentieth-century prophet David Koresh living in provincial Texas both believed themselves and their disciples to be participants in history's endgame. No matter how minor (or major) their place in the social structure of the time and no matter their disenfranchisement from social, economic, and political power, apocalyptists believe themselves to belong to the elect and to be participants in a cosmic struggle. It is not surprising, therefore, that the second half of the twentieth century witnessed an increase in apocalyptic beliefs.

Throughout the last decade of the twentieth century and into the twenty-first, as the technomediated world prepared for the turn of the second millennium of the common era into the third, millennialist aspirations and apocalyptic anxieties affected intellectuals, the media, and groups of doomsday believers and extremists. With the dissolution of the former Soviet bloc in Eastern Europe and the demise of the Soviet Union, neoconservatives like Francis Fukuyama were proclaiming the decisive victory of capitalism over communism; in *The End of History and the Last Man*, Fukuyama announced that history had entered its last stage, the triumph of liberal democracy. However, the "end of ideology" was a premature declaration as a variety of religious beliefs have asserted themselves nationally and internationally. Agents of the United States federal government in 1993 sought the arrest of David Koresh, leader of a breakaway branch of the Davidian millennial reform movement within the Seventh-Day Adventist Church. The armed standoff between the Branch Davidians and federal forces resulted in the deaths of several federal agents and scores of Davidian believers. In 1995, the Japanese Aum Shinrikyo cult carried out a sarin gas attack on the Tokyo subway (culminating a series of attacks on its perceived enemies) motivated by its millennialist belief in its struggle against a global conspiracy of evil. Two suicidal millennialist cults became news in the 1990s. Members of the Order of the Solar Temple committed suicide in Quebec and Switzerland in 1994 followed by other members in France in 1995 and again in

Quebec in 1997; history was coming to an end, they prophesied, and they were leaving the world to an apocalyptic catastrophe. In 1997, thirty-nine Heaven's Gate cult members under the leadership of Marshall Applewhite committed suicide because their "physical containers" were no longer needed; they interpreted the appearance of the Hale-Bopp comet that year as a sign of the end. However, millennialist anticipation was not the monopoly of marginal cults; the Western world, particularly the computer-dependent United States, was preoccupied with the per-ceived threat of the so-called Y2K bug, a computer programming anomaly that threatened complex infrastructures of communication, transporta-tion, finance, and commerce. In response, right-wing survivalists retreated to isolated but well-stocked rural enclaves to sit out the ensuing social chaos. However, technology planning, massive investment in information technologies and computer programming, and diligence can be said to have prevented most of the anticipated problems, but it did not prevent considerable media hype imagining what might occur at midnight on December 31, 1999. Diligence also precipitated the border arrest on December 14 of a suspected terrorist attempting to enter the United States from Canada with explosives in his vehicle; convicted in a millennial plot to attack the Los Angeles airport, Ahmed Ressam later provided testimony concerning the operations of Osama bin Laden's Al Quaida terrorist cells.[4]

It is reasonable to suggest that Islamic fundamentalisms, of the sort that probably impelled the attacks on September 11, 2001 (as well as those before and since), draw from the same well of Judeo-Christian apocalypticism, and similarly invite contradictory responses. At least it feels apocalyptic to the West. Robert Jay Lifton has suggested that "to many people close to it, in New York and Washington, [the attacks felt] like some version of the end of the world. That is how people in Hiroshima felt." By situating those attacks within the horizon of other "unthinkable" events of the twentieth century, Lifton encourages us to believe that the "initial sense of the world ending can be altered and transformed into various expressions of rebuilding and reconstruction," precisely the kind of agency that the AIDS crisis has summoned. In contrast, Michael Hardt and Antonio Negri's *Empire* presents an oracular vision of maraud-ing hordes advancing upon industrialized, nation-state empires. It feels to them less like the beginning of the twenty-first century and more like the beginning of the fifth, a globalism that strikes back at the empire. Ben-jamin Barber has made a similar binary opposition out of Islamic militants' resistance to global capitalism in his *Jihad vs. McWorld: How Globalism and Tribalism Are Reshaping the World*. As long as Islamo-Arabic dominance in the Middle East prevailed, *jihad* could be generally understood as a spiritual struggle. It is not surprising, therefore, that following European colonization of the Middle East and the collapse of the Ottoman Empire, an Islamic militancy emerged that literalized *jihad* in much the same what that some Christians imagine Armageddon: a final military battle of good over evil. Not far from the Pentagon in Northern Virginia, students in the Islamic Saudi Academy learn from a textbook, according a report in the *Washington Post*, that Judgment Day will come when Jesus returns to earth, breaks the cross and converts people to Islam, and faithful Moslems hunt Jews. Rather than the apocalypse of ideology, we are witnessing a new stage in the globalization of ideology, ideology without borders.[5]

Global epidemic disease continues to evoke apocalyptic responses. One aspect of increasingly global economic and social structures is expanded human mobility by improved travel technologies, which to an epidemiologist reads "vectors of transmission." This presents us with the prospect of worldwide, not simply local, epidemics, whose exoticism and the incapacity of public health services even in the industrialized world are ripe for the apocalyptic signifier "plague." HIV has become globalized as a result of transportation networks, despite its prevention and treatment strategies' being well documented. More alarming, perhaps, are diseases transmitted by animal. The English foot-and-mouth epidemic of 2001 was commonly characterized as "apocalyptic," at least for the English who witnessed burning heaps of culled animal carcasses that dotted their normally pastoral English countryside. The emergence and proliferation in the Eastern United States of West Nile Virus (whose name says it all, an evocation of a biblical plague) captured media attention in 2000, reintroducing that ancient disease vector, the mosquito, at a time when eco-apocalypse in the form of global warming was accompanied by the proliferation of mosquitoes. Bioterrorism has loomed large recently following the handful of anthrax-laced letters (a common animal illness here deployed in a relatively low-tech fashion) that succeeded briefly in shutting down the legislative branches of the United States and disrupting news media. Anthrax is generally considered to be a difficult disease to contract and usually easy to treat, but even it has tested the resources of public and private health systems that have been made leaner (and meaner) during a decade of reductions in public funding and of "managed care" in the United States. Journalist

Laurie Garrett, who has made something of a career pronouncing Cassandra-like prophecies of infectious disease judgment, suggests that, even in industrialized nations with national health systems, infectious diseases would become unmanageable, her findings published in such books as *Betrayal of Trust: The Collapse of Global Public Health* and *The Coming Plague: Newly Emerging Diseases in a World Out of Balance*. Apocalypse sells books, though one is now less inclined to dismiss the rhetoric of the unthinkable after witnessing the collapse of the World Trade Center towers.[6]

Africa is generally believed to be the source of HIV, but in the imagination of the industrialized world it is also the source of a variety of apocalyptically conceived plagues. Isolated outbreaks of Ebola virus and other hemorraghic fevers are regularly reported in Western media. This anxiety about Africa was evident in the 1995 film *Outbreak*, in which actors Dustin Hoffman and Cuba Gooding, Jr. are depicted fighting a viral epidemic carried by an infected African monkey that escapes in Northern California. If these are exceptional and rare infectious diseases, the epidemiology of African AIDS is staggering in its prevalence: at the turn of the millennium, of the world's 36 million HIV infected, 25 million lived in Africa. The reasons for this devastation are many: poverty, lack of sanitation and health care, migrancy, the prevalence of drug use and sex work, the frequency of rape, civil war, folk healing beliefs and practices (such as the one asserting that having sex with a virgin is a cure for AIDS), among others. Complicit in the catastrophe has been the indifference and inaction of the wealthy industrialized world, which failed to supply Africans with the programs and resources that had been proven to prevent and manage HIV transmission and infection. At the same time, the inaction of African governments is also to blame. The toll in South African, newly freed from apartheid rule in 1993, has been the most distressing; it has the largest number of HIV-positive citizens in the world. The apartheid National Party had used fear of AIDS in its campaign against the African National Congress; what had initially been stigmatized as a "Gay Plague" suddenly became "Black Death" with racist images of hypersexual black men fueling white anxieties. However, upon the end of apartheid, black majority leaders were in no better position to confront the epidemic, and Nelson Mandela's successor in the presidency, Thabo Mbeki, has questioned the medical consensus about HIV and resisted providing government funds for making antiviral drugs available to pregnant women, choosing instead to call for moral reform. If there is a population that deserves the right to configure AIDS in apocalyptic terms, sub-Saharan Africans are it, but the trope is also used for the same demonizing purposes in Africa as in the United States. Robert Mugabe, president of Zimbabwe, frequently characterized AIDS as a message from God calling people to moral reform and repeatedly targeted homosexuality as a national threat.[7]

Because my own continuing work for twenty years has been devoted to educational praxis and grassroots activism, the preoccupations of this study have been the material conditions involved in the production of apocalyptic tropes and their effects, the cultural or semiosic work they perform. Perhaps in part because I am also the product of an American pragmatic culture, I have been more interested in critical praxis than in critical theory, although I realize even the instability of that binarism. While theoretical analysis has been helpful at strategic moments of this study, I have been far more inclined toward an analysis that distinguishes which liberatory practices work within the horizon of given historical circumstances. In that respect I have suggested that while apocalyptic tropes representing AIDS have had tactical efficacy, their strategic usefulness has never been more than provisional and has often been dangerous. The same discourse that mobilizes group solidarity also calcifies communities into rigid identities or stereotypes that deny or resist the very fluidity of "identity." The provisional nature of one set of material conditions makes yesterday's effective practices useless today.

Effective classroom praxis under the aegis of advocacy pedagogy clearly should be grounded in the cultural conditions of students and their analysis of their own and others' cultures. Among other things, now more than twenty years into the epidemic, many students know someone who has or has died from HIV-related illness. My students have grieved for a friend, brother, or parent. One twenty-something student of mine left the college after visiting the Names Project Quilt in Washington, DC, because, as he told me, he became overwhelmed by the grief represented there that he could no longer imagine going to school to prepare for a career. In contrast, another began a college education because pharmaceutical advances have given him a future. Their responses are contradictory, but they illustrate the kinds of paradoxes this epidemic generates even in North America. In Third World nations, the contradictions are even more stark. Classroom practices need to examine, but not adjudicate among, these important paradoxes. In the classroom we must resist the American cultural tendency to marginalize or commodify AIDS and instead advocate for critical analysis and discursive practices that undermine binary oppositions.

"AIDS education" particularly has undergone a thorough revision in the last few years. During the first decade of the epidemic, activists and health workers found the construction of some binarisms tactically useful in treatment and infection prevention, such as safe sex/unsafe sex or HIV-negative/HIV-positive. Later critiques of these efforts, however, have questioned their continuing efficacy. By the early 1990s risk-reduction education in many places had dismantled the safe/unsafe binarism in favor of a triune "safe/possibly-safe/unsafe," but not without controversy. Robin Gorna, for example, points out that Britain's Terrence Higgins Trust (THT), an AIDS service organization (ASO), was demonized at the 1992 International Conference on AIDS (held in Amsterdam) by ACT UP members, many of whom did not even know that the organization was an ASO. At a "zap" (impromptu demonstration) against THT, members of New York's Gay Men's Health Crisis (GMHC) and Lesbian AIDS Project (LAP) insisted that the women of THT attend an evening meeting:

> In the small room, crammed with over sixty women, we were systematically ignored. The meeting was fascinating, with an *evangelical* feel. There was repeated '*testimony*' from HIV-positive lesbians, all from New York, all from LAP. Early on, one of the women started to shout, 'demanding' that lesbians with HIV in the room come out, protesting that their silence was killing her by reinforcing invisibility and isolation. She insisted that she 'knew' that there were lesbians present who were HIV-positive but keeping quiet. She was insistent, angry and aggressive. What was so telling about this meeting was the way in which the women polarized into '*right-thinking*' lesbians (pro-latex) and '*wrong-thinking*' (THT and closeted HIV-positive lesbians). The antagonism and lack of discussion was [sic] as sharp as in the porn wars and SM debates [emphasis mine].

Of even greater concern more recently has been the alarming increase in the numbers of formerly HIV-negative gay men who have "seroconverted," a public health euphemism applied to people's engaging in behavior that results in HIV infection with the consequent development of viral antibodies in the blood. The poster child of this disturbing epidemiological trend may be the neoconservative homosexual pundit, Andrew Sullivan, who "seroconverted" in the 1990s and was later accused of soliciting "barebacking" sex (i.e., anal sex without using condoms) on the Internet. In a 1997 essay in the (London) *Independent on Sunday* entitled "When Plagues End: Notes on the Twilight of an Epidemic" Sullivan opined that

"When you have spent several years girding yourself for the possibility of death, it is not so easy to gird yourself instead for the possibility of life. What you expect to greet with euphoria of victory comes instead like the slow withdrawal of an excuse. And you resist it. The intensity with which you had learned to approach each day turns into a banality." The emergence of pharmaceutical advertising in mainstream media may have contributed to this inadvertently. The young men in ads for antivirals and protease inhibitors (and the drugs needed to combat the host of side effects of antivirals and protease inhibitors) are sexy and athletic. You want them; you want to be them. Got AIDS? We have a pill for that now. David Román has suggested that the media attention paid to gay HIV-positive men has left a vacuum in the representation of gay HIV-negative men who experience themselves as unrepresentable, if you will, the serostatus that is not one. Noting the frequent hostility to the suggestion that HIV-negative gay men need support to maintain their status, psychologist Walt Odets has observed that, "being uninfected . . . entails special problems of personal and social identity and, often, a feeling of disenfranchisement from the minority community that has provided the uninfected gay man with acceptance and a sense of who he is and where he belongs. For these reasons, being uninfected is often fraught with conflict and ambivalence." Similarly, Eric Rofes pointed to the grief and alienation gay men experience in the context of catastrophic loss as a cause of their risk taking, despite their familiarity with HIV transmission vectors. Rofes called for "regeneration" in the gay male world by dismantling our exclusively rigid, binaristic identities with AIDS and homosexuality. Ironically, even in the very clinical discourse of AIDS, we return again and again to the religious discourse that saturates North American society: "right/wrong," "conversion," "regeneration," "testimony," "evangelical."[8]

Similarly, forms of gay, lesbian, bisexual and transgendered activism must break free of a rigid identity politics while they also dismantle the assimilationist/separatist opposition. Although tactically useful, identity politics share a metonymic brittleness with apocalyptic discourse. Categories of identity belie the complexities and multiplicities of subjectivity while they often prevent tactically advantageous alliances. Roman Catholics in New York are a case in point. The tendency of many AIDS activists to characterize all Catholics based on the activists' perceptions of the Catholic hierarchy is blind to the prevalence of sexual dissent within the church, as the priest-sociologist Andrew Greeley has frequently pointed out. Moreover, as Chris Bull and John Gallagher observe in *Perfect Enemies: The*

Religious Right, the Gay Movement, and the Politics of the 1990s, lesbian and gay activists have been as determined as Christian fundamentalists to demonize their ideological opponents (although less virulently), with the result of utterly polarizing any public discussion of sexuality. In the 1992 United States presidential election, Americans declined the Republican Party's invitation (delivered by Pat Buchanan) to march onward toward Armageddon in a righteous culture war against liberals, feminists, and homosexuals.[9] Conservative apocalyptic vehemence went underground, nurtured by the likes of Rev. Fred Phelps, the Kansas preacher who appears uninvited at funerals of AIDS patients or of victims of hate crimes while carrying signs that read, "Fags Doom Nations," as well as networks of hate groups that proliferate using Web sites and shortwave radio (such as Brother R. G. Stair of the Overcomer Ministry, whose apocalyptic commentary has been documented by the Southern Poverty Law Center: "The last two Gay Pride Days have resulted in an awesome earthquake that shook the entire Western area of the country and a flood that devastated the entire Midwest. . . . You mark my word, ladies and gentlemen, they are going to bring total destruction to a pagan, immoral, un-Godly, wicked, sin-loving nation such as ours"). Eventually, smarter religious conservatives shifted their exoteric discourse from the oracles of the jeremiad to the rhetoric of compassion: Hate the sin but love the sinner. However, out of the wreckage of New York's World Trade Center and Arlington, Virginia's Pentagon building, Pat Robertson and Jerry Falwell pronounced that the terrorist attacks were the result of God's lifting his protection because the United States had tolerated homosexuals, feminists, and the American Civil Liberties Union. Later, the Tulsa, Oklahoma, Church of God Outreach Ministries took out a quarter-page advertisement in the October 26, 2001 *USA Today,* in which the church answered its own question—Why Is American the Target of Terrorists?—with the answer: "The terror, the death, the pain will continue as we have failed to protect the unborn, we have tolerated and encouraged homosexual relationships and we have found pleasure in every kind of sexual depravity known to man." As my psychiatrist regularly reminds me, When under stress, we regress. Subsequently, contributor appeals that I received from the National Gay and Lesbian Taskforce and the Human Rights Campaign have warned me of our impending doom at the hands of the Religious Right. Apocalypse is good for everybody's fund raising.[10]

   The dichotomy of assimilation and separatism has also hampered gay and lesbian activism for decades. The politics of sameness or difference are never so simple or unalloyed as that opposition supposes they are. American cultural politics are historically a precarious alchemy of assimilation and separatism that is never a steady state. There is even a semantic ambiguity within the physiological trope "assimilation," which means "to ingest" as in an organism's ingesting of nutrients. However, who "ingests" whom in cultural assimilation is never quite clear since cultural dominance and cultural marginality are similarly unstable categories. Does the "marginal" culture "ingest" the "dominant" culture or vice versa? Perhaps more accurately, to use an alchemical metaphor, both are amalgamated. While the mass culture celebrity of television's *Will and Grace* or *Queer Eye for the Straight Guy* seems, to some commentators, to have marked gay assimilation into the American mainstream, those programs did not protect Matthew Shepard from frontier thugs nor do they afford gay, lesbian, bisexual, or transgendered people the legal or medical parity they deserve. Perhaps the only advance we can claim is that there is now widespread disdain for Christian fundamentalists' apocalyptic demonizing of queer people. However, for combative gay gadfly Daniel Harris, such mainstream assimilation is itself an apocalypse, as reflected in the title of his 1997 book: *The Rise and Fall of Gay Culture*. Now a "lifestyle" with its own brands, Harris contends, Gay™ is just another commodity and we have witnessed the Twilight of the Fabulous.[11]

I have argued throughout this study that sexual dissidents and AIDS activists had in large measure assimilated and rescripted Western religious apocalypticism, often doing so, however, while repudiating traditional religion. Although many urban activists and significant queer culture figures are not religious, the same cannot be said for millions of gay, lesbian, bisexual, and transgendered people in the United States (the most overtly religious of the Western nations). Paradoxically, the principle of the separation of church and state has produced in the United States a public religiosity that is unparalleled in other industrialized countries. This phenomenon has been variously called our "secular religion" and the "American religion," which Harold Bloom has characterized as a form of Gnosticism.[12] In the United States, the dialectical materialism or positivism of many gay activists has tended to view religious or spiritual discourse as false ideology or psychological illusion, thus inevitably an obstacle to liberation or well-being. However, critical of both gay mainstream assimilationism and political Marxism, Mitch Walker, whose work has influenced Douglas Sadownick and others, carves out a space for those drawn to mythic spiritualities: "We want to seek out our vision, which we sense contains a unique and necessary contribution to the freedom of humanity . . . key to the evolution of humanity to a new stage of being." This seems like old essentialism writ large, or at least, writ New Age, but it is an assessment held by several important figures in queer leadership. Judy Grahn, author of the gay cultural history *Another Mother Tongue*, contends that "gay people have a history—continual, interwoven, and worldwide—[and] what is more remarkable and will probably preoccupy me for the rest of my life is the understanding that gay people have a social purpose." Grahn's attitude was anticipated by Harry Hay, godfather of queer activism, who in the early years of the Mattachine Society (1950–53) formulated the questions that Douglas Sadownick and Ian Young have recently recovered: "Who are we gay people? Where do we come from, in history and in anthropology, and where have we been? What are we for?"[13]

Not surprisingly, when many gay and lesbian people began to confront the limit situation of an epidemic disease that medical technologies could not control, they frequently resorted to the discourse of a dimension of ultimacy.[14] For example, in a series of conversations published as *Muses from Chaos and Ash: AIDS, Artists, and Art*, Andréa R. Vaucher elicited responses from HIV-positive artists on a variety of concerns, including spirituality. Playwright and performance artist Reza Abdoh suggested:

> AIDS has created a landscape in which the body and the spirit and the politic of the body and the spirit can be examined, reshaped, restructured, destroyed, and reformed. I think it's important for us as a people who are not embracing the status quo to discover our own road to what you might want to call redemption or salvation. It has nothing whatsoever to do with the Judeo-Christian idea of salvation or redemption. It has to do with a certain kind of peace that you find within yourself and you transmit, hopefully, through a generous act to your community. I think the queer community has managed to come to some kind of an understanding of that need for discovery.

Having undergone his own vision quest after a fast-lane career working with Andy Warhol's *Interview*, writer Mark Matousek observed:

> Instigating conversations about spirituality in the presence of suffering, I learned, is to risk vulgarity, to miss the point, to literalize what is by its nature subtle, personal, and silent. As Joe Miller, a PWA living in

New York, puts it, "Spirituality is like sex: The ones who really have it don't talk about it." There are two primary reasons for resistance to the "S" word. The first concerns the attitude of organized religion toward homosexuals, who continue to dominate the AIDS community. . . . [and] certain factions of the New Age movement, whose saccharine philosophy is the second major obstacle to spirit among individuals groping with the gritty reality of AIDS.[15]

The result of this explicit attention to spiritual discourse has been a profusion of publications about queer spiritualities. Mainstream publishers, popular publications, and even academic journals have circulated a wide variety of discussions of sacred homosex. For example, the June 29, 1993 issue of the *Village Voice* (the Gay Pride issue, which that year followed on the heels of the national gay, lesbian, and bisexual march in Washington, DC, earlier in the spring), included a series of articles under Richard Goldstein's lead, "Faith, Hope, and Sodomy: Gay Liberation Embarks on a Vision Quest."[16] Even more remarkable than this series from the typically iconoclastic *Voice* was a series in *Frontiers*, a Los Angeles publication that usually sports a big, buff hunk on its cover. The September 10, 1993 issue featured pieces on "The Gay and Lesbian Religious Movement in America," "The Spirit of AIDS," and "Catching Up 2 Queer Theology."[17] In the Fall 1996 issue of *The Harvard Gay & Lesbian Review*, editor Richard Schneider, Jr., collected a series of articles, book excerpts, and reviews under the rubric "Homo Spiritualis," confessing that, "The idea for an issue on religion and spirituality was suggested by the sheer weight of manuscripts that I received in a curiously short span of time last winter. Perhaps a more religious person than I would have found in this confluence a deeper meaning than merely, 'Time to do an issue on religion.'"[18] To discern "deeper meaning" in a "confluence" of the discrete: Schneider admits that he is (with a nod to Weber) " 'religiously unmusical' " and although he may not know the tune, he nonetheless recognizes the lyrics.

The postmodern condition—the absence of a single monolithic, stable "condition" apprehended under a master narrative—seems particularly haunted by memories of that music and traces of those lyrics. In *Post-Modernism and the Social Sciences: Insights, Inroads, and Intrusions*, Pauline Marie Rosenau suggests that postmodernity, particularly in "New Age" sensibilities, finds mystical or spiritual discourse appealing in its suspicion of modernist rationalism.[19] Andrew Wernick's assessment runs along similar lines, alluding to the apocalyptic desires stimulated in part as the third millennium of the Common Era approached:

> At the moment of death, so it is said, your whole life flashes before you. No surprise, then, as we glide—comfortably, some of us, yet dystopically— towards the turn of the second millennium, a movement shadowed by foreboding, but even more by the collective sense of becoming-dead, of—socially speaking—entropic dissolution, that contemporary western culture should be saturated by nostalgia for what is irredeemably past. Nor that it should be haunted—or rather revisited—by archaic meta- phors that have welled up from our sedimented pre-industrial imaginary. It is in such terms, at least, that we might plausibly account for the recently revived interest in religion—an interest manifest not only in popular fun- damentalism, but also, and more paradoxically, in the preoccupation with the mystical, the spiritual and the religious that has surfaced within the new postmodernist (and therefore post-post-Enlightenment) theoreticians of the secular intelligentsia.[20]

This reflection comes from Wernick's discussion of theological themes in Jean Baudrillard's *America*. In a later text, *The Illusion of the End*, Baudrillard himself suggests that postmodern religiosity is the product of fin de siècle grief and rage:

> We used to ask what might come after the orgy—mourning or melan- cholia? Doubtless neither, but an interminable clean-up of all the vicis- situdes of modern history and its processes of liberation (of peoples, sex, dreams, art and the unconscious—in short, of all that makes up the orgy of our times), in an atmosphere dominated by the apocalyptic presentiment that all this is coming to an end. Rather than pressing forward and taking flight into the future, we prefer the retrospective apocalypse, and a blanket revisionism.

While dismissing melancholia here, later in the same text Baudrillard asserts that "the new labour power, which has emerged in this fin de siècle, is mourning power. . . . As something which has failed, this work of mourning is interminable." After AIDS we yearn nostalgically for absent pleasures, including the pleasures of spirituality. Is spiritual dis- course always, then, only the recycling of trashed ideologies? Can it ever now be more or other than an "attempt to escape the apocalypse of the virtual" which is "the last of our utopian desires"?[21] Is the postmodern "condition" the second apocalypse of spirituality following its first apocalypse in modernism's critique of religion as false ideology and illusion?

I want to wager that it is not—and that it is. In naming this chapter, "(In)conclusion," I am attempting to map what for me is the post-Christian (and more personally post-Catholic and postmetaphysical) trajectory of my own life and, by doing so, to make room not for indecision or for contradiction, but for paradox and "inconclusion" as the "uncertainty field" (in a Heisenbergian sense) in which we pulsate, the performance that cannot be stabilized into a freeze frame, and whose significance is knowable only as an excess, boundless signification, the free play of signifiers; or to use American theologian John S. Dunne's definition of *mystery*, "not unintelligibility but inexhaustible intelligibility."[22] Carl Raschke urges us to consider this:

> The differend is the antonym of the referent; but is also something much more, and far stranger, than what Paul Ricoeur and others have termed as "plurisignificative," the unlimited semiosis that characterizes fluid and allusive language. The differend is the pure unvocalizable that quivers not only at the boundaries of discourse, but at the fringes of existence. Like the Heideggerian *nihil*, Lyotard's *differend* is both limit and horizon. It is the "line" circumscribing signification beyond which a new and more fundamental occasion for "semiophany" becomes possible. The end of the age of the sign, disclosed in the *differend*, in the silence, is at the same time an overture to what is genuinely postmodern, understood at last as a total presence, an eschatological fullness, a *parousia*—after the fashion of Heidegger—of the very sign-universe.[23]

What I want to recommend is the fruitfulness of an exploration of spiritual signification that is more concerned with the semiosic plane (the cultural work that signification performs) than with the mimetic plane (its claims to represent "reality"). I am urging that scholars and cultural critics can pay respectful attention to religious discourses without needing to reduce or to adopt them.

Many African Americans and feminists in the past century have had to construct a praxis of political spirituality out of the immediate threats to their bodies. The late Audre Lorde, a self-described "Black Lesbian Feminist," articulated both the resistance to and the necessity for mystical praxis:

> As women, we have come to distrust that power which rises from our deepest and non-rational knowledge. We have been warned against it

all our lives by the male world, which values this depth of feeling enough to keep women around in order to exercise it in the service of men, but which fears this same depth too much to examine the possibilities of it within themselves. So women are maintained at a distant/inferior position to be psychically milked, much the same way ants maintain colonies of aphids to provide a life-giving substance for their masters. But the erotic offers a well of replenishing and provocative force to the woman who does not fear its revelation, nor succumb to the belief that sensation is enough.[24]

Likewise, Beverly Wildung Harrison and Carter Heyward were intrepid enough to use the term "transcendence," which they characterized as "the wellspring of religious intuition and spiritual resourcefulness" and which is nothing less than "the power to cross over from self to other," a crossing over that can occur in sex.[25] Karin Lofthus Carrington made a similar observation: "It became clear that through my experience of loving women and being loved by them, eros had called me beyond my separativeness, beyond those constricting separate chambers in my own heart. Eros has a way of doing that. And the love of women for women does it in a particular way." Transcendental discourses can be understood as ways of resisting master narratives, such as reductionism, in favor of the inexhaustibility of human experience.[26]

AIDS work in American communities of color—historically marginalized from adequate health care and susceptible to homophobia—will succeed only insofar as it leverages the discourses of spirituality on behalf of the infected and the affected. Frequently in these communities, the spiritual is the political. Unfortunately, a decade and a half of church moralizing in those communities only delayed this work, and they now reap the whirlwind. As early as 1989, Calu Lester and Larry Saxxon had characterized this delay "within communities of black and brown people" as allowing "a virtual time bomb to slowly but steadily tick away" and placed the blame at the feet of leaders in communities of color as well as the AIDS establishment. In 1991, one African American minister, Rev. Dr. W.C. Champion, presiding elder of the Christian Methodist Episcopal Church of Dallas, Texas, observed that "The Black church needs to deal with the apparent ignorance of AIDS that is so prevalent within the Black church and community. The Black church needs to deal with the theological issues of AIDS and answer questions members and pastors have." In many African American com-

munities and churches, AIDS was long viewed as a white or homosexual problem, and in those congregations married men and women
were assumed to be heterosexual, which impeded education and prevention efforts. In her study of religious minorities' apocalyptic AIDS
discourses, Susan Palmer found that some members of the Nation of
Islam believe that African AIDS is the result of CIA germ warfare
experiments using Africans as research subjects. By the turn of the
millennium the Centers for Disease Control and Prevention (CDC)
were reporting that more than half of new AIDS cases among gay men
were African American or Latino men. Stigmatization of homosexuality
among people of color has been so persistent, according to Dr. Helen
Gayle, a CDC director, that nearly one-quarter of African American
men and one-sixth of Latin men who are having sex with other men
still classify themselves as "heterosexual."[27]

Both Douglas Sadownick and Ian Young have proposed their own
analyses of North American gay male culture in regard to spiritual praxis,
which I have discussed in the previous chapter. Among them have emerged
a crowd of other voices.[28] Although it is intellectually safe to dismiss this
prolific spiritual discourse as nostalgic, ideologically erroneous, or illusory
(and this reaction is particularly characteristic of academic critics), I would
urge that such a dismissal is modernist reductionism insofar as dismissal
would claim the status of master narrative over what is clearly in American society a valuable way of composing meaning. A component of
popular culture, religious discourse deserves attention on its own merits
and within its own self-understandings, without being dismissed out of
hand as oppression or alienation. As Carl Raschke has pointed out:

> A social semiotics needs no longer to presuppose that signification
> *equals* oppression, that is invariably a vertical imposition of symbol-
> controllers upon the mass, but that it may also be a kind of *cri de coeur*
> of the disenfranchised. The horizontal dissemination of sign-perfor-
> mances through a 'decentered' popular culture does not necessarily
> legitimate either their moral or ontological character, but reframes their
> purpose, primarily in terms of the categories of regimentation, subver-
> sion, 'ceremonial' articulation and ideological oscillations. According to
> the sociologist Erving Goffman . . . the "commercialism" of so much
> popular culture can best be considered a complex set of typifications
> that are not so far distant from ritualized, everyday language and
> behaviour. Sign-events cluster around 'displays,' which in turn coalesce

around different social codings, not to mention *codings of difference*, may or may not be co-ordinate with the insignia of class.

The sheer mass of published materials on queer spirituality, not to mention a range of other performative practices like meditation, spiritual reading, ritual, and the like, claims our interested attention. Moreover, since "sexuality and popular religion . . . cannot be disentangled from each other because of their very 'carnivality' (in Eco's sense), or 'incarnality' from a broader semiotic perspective,"[29] religious theory might acknowledge how it is entangled in discourse and semiotic theory, how it is entangled in mystery, that is, inexhaustible intelligibility.

Throughout this study I have urged cautious attention to and suspicion of apocalypticism, and now I would extend that caution to apocalyptic mysticism. In a collection for the Catholic Paulist Press Classics of Western Spirituality series, Bernard McGinn, the preminent North American scholar of apocalypticism, writes of an "apocalyptic spirituality" by which he means "the ways in which apocalypticism affects the believer and his actions," particularly when the believers understand themselves as people in crisis. What is unspoken here is the way the apocalypticism of the believers and their actions affect others, especially since, as McGinn points out, "the apocalypticist [sic] might be better described as one on the lookout for crisis . . . [and] more in need of a religious structure within which to absorb and give meaning to the anxieties that always accompany existence and change." This caution has been necessary in light of American discourse on homosexual desires and on AIDS over the past thirty years.[30]

It has been easy to produce a Christian fundamentalist Other whose apocalyptic discourse demonizes queer desires—along with demonizing many other signifiers of postmodern fluidity. In the long term, however, this approach creates a hall of mirrors whose infinite regression reproduces endless distortions. Queer folk have been producers of apocalyptic panic, and not simply as the purveyors of what is sometimes called "secular" apocalypses. Poet Mark Doty lamented in the essay "Is There a Future?":

> My Christian grandmother . . . used to read me passages from the Book of Revelation and talk about the imminence of the Last Days. . . . By the time I was an adolescent I was quickly outgrowing religion when another sense of the apocalyptic replaced it, the late sixties' faith in the imminence of revolution. . . . One sort of apocalyptic scenario has re-

placed another: endings ecological or nuclear, scenarios of depleted ozone or global starvation or, finally, epidemic. All my life I've lived with a future which constantly diminishes but never vanishes. Apocalypse is played out now in a personal scale; it is not in the sky above us but in our bed.

In *AIDS and Its Metaphors* Susan Sontag described the West's condition similarly: "With the inflation of apocalyptic rhetoric has come the increasing unreality of the apocalypse. A permanent modern scenario: apocalypse looms . . . and it doesn't occur. And it still looms. We seem to be in the throes of one of the modern kinds of apocalypse. . . . Apocalypse is now a long-running serial: not 'Apocalypse Now' but 'Apocalypse From Now On.' " Eternally deferred, this apocalypse gives us the panic without the spectacle of closure. Is panic the spiritual state of postmodernity?[31]

Ironically, two gay writers touched by AIDS and devoted to mysticism seem also to be susceptible to an apocalyptic spirituality. In *Sex, Death, and Enlightenment*, a memoir of life in New York's fast lanes, Mark Matousek rendered his first encounter with a man who would become his lover and spiritual mentor, whom he interviewed for an issue of Andy Warhol's *Interview*:

> Alexander looked me straight in the eyes. . . . "The world is much worse than it's ever been. We're at the end of an entire cycle of history, you know. . . . The apocalypse. . . . How much time do we have, anyway? Twenty years at the most? Everyone must now admit that the end is in sight. 'Work now, for the night is coming,' it says in Ecclesiastes."

Later in the same conversation, "Alexander" told Mark, " 'The world is on fire. The things that genuinely matter—truth, beauty, honor, spirit—are all in ruins. And here you sit, a young man obviously at some kind of crossroads, at the very core of the inferno, slaving for the devil himself." This characterization then prompted Matousek's apocalyptic imagination:

> Again, he took my breath away. How many times had I watched Warhol waft by my office, ghostlike, his sharp dead eyes surveying his kingdom, and felt an actual chill pass through me? How often had I secretly wondered whether Andy wasn't really the Antichrist—not Andy the man, of course, but Andy the symbol—a clever fraud feeding off the entrails of capitalism like a hyena? How often had I wondered, finally,

what this equation said about me, and whether I hadn't made a pact
with the devil by becoming one of his lackeys.[32]

"Alexander" of this memoir was actually writer and mystic Andrew Harvey,
who in an interview with Mark Thompson in *Gay Soul* characterized
AIDS as "a kind of training ground for the apocalypse. I feel that those
people who are dying of AIDS are going through in their bodies what is
actually happening to the earth. . . . AIDS is a challenge to all of us to
become as awake and enlightened as possible, to live as intensely and
presently in love as possible."[33] In a text later coauthored with Matousek,
Harvey insisted that, "This is not an apocalyptic scenario, not a 'scenario'
at all, in fact. It is where we are; it is what is happening; it is terrifying,
and anyone not in a trance of denial knows it. No amount of wishful
thinking and sophisticated drawing of pseudohistorical parallels can make
this agony go away."[34]

Harvey's mimetic claims trumped his semiosic claims; his voice was
not simply hortatory but oracular. He insisted that he was describing
"where we are . . . what is happening" rather than employing hyperbole
for rhetorical ends. But Harvey's apocalyptic sublime transfixes us, para-
lyzing both thinking and acting. As with every apocalyptist, he giveth
and he taketh away, because while his admonition asks us to change, the
immensity announces that it is too late. One product of such discourse,
as Lee Quinby points out, is that it displaces forms of analysis:

> At stake here are the relationships between power, truth, ethics, and
> apocalypse. In attempting to represent the unrepresentable, the un-
> knowable—the End, or death par excellence—apocalyptic writings are
> a quintessential technology of power/knowledge. They promise the defeat
> of death, at least for the obedient who deserve everlasting life, and the
> prolonged agony of destruction for those who have not obeyed the Law
> of the Father. One does not have to succumb to apocalyptic eschatology
> to understand why end-time propensities imperil democracy: the apoca-
> lyptic tenet of preordained history disavows questionings of received
> truth, discredits skepticism, and disarms challengers of the status quo.[35]

Historically, experiential mysticisms have tended to absorb ambiguity
and to resist authoritarian claims of dogmatic institutional religion. Individuals and collectives who devote themselves to the "plurisignificative,"
the "differend," and "semiophany," who read inexhaustible intelligibility
and paradox into problem and contradiction, will likewise resist the master

narratives of dogmatism in favor of the fragmented, dispersed, and local. It is not a novel paradox, but was described by one seventeenth-century Puritan apocalyptist, John Milton: "We do not see that, while we still affect by all means a rigid external formality, we may as soon fall again into a gross conforming stupidity, a stark and dead congealment of wood and hay and stubble, forced and frozen together, which is more to the sudden degenerating . . . than many subdichotomies of petty schisms."[36]

In conclusion, . . . there is none, though that will not stop apocalyptists from imagining the imminent eschaton. Apocalypticism (even the secular variety), like the poor, thou shalt always have with you. The same may be said for religious belief and practice generally. This assertion is discomforting for many academic scholars and cultural critics; our methods are empirical and we tend to hold, almost as an article of faith, to the secularization thesis, the faith of our Enlightenment and Victorian intellectual fathers (and mothers). Our inclination is to approach religion in reductionistic ways, as false ideology or neurosis, for example, and by doing so we impose our own (equally dogmatic) master narrative. However, religious discourse has not retreated from the advance of science, technology, and social science; indeed, the opposite has occurred, both in industrialized nations (particularly the United States) and in the developing world. Two centuries of oracular utterances about the apocalypse of religion and the imminent rationalist millennium constitute the secularist's faith. The task of the scholar and the cultural critic in the twenty-first century will be to acknowledge the semiosic functions of religious discourses, and, without abandoning our own commitments to the study of material cultural conditions, to question and resist those discourses' mimetic claims. We can acknowledge the value of religious discourse without endorsing its claims to represent the real.

Notes

NOTES TO CHAPTER ONE

1. Dr. Lawrence Mass, a gay physician, was the author of the first article to appear in a gay newspaper, "Disease Rumors Largely Unfounded," *New York Native* May 18–31, 1981, 7. Lawrence Altman was the author of the second, "Rare Cancer Seen in 41 Homosexuals," *New York Times*, July 3, 1981, 20. Jerry Falwell is best known as a television evangelist, pastor of Liberty Baptist Church, founder of Liberty College in Lynchburg, Virginia, and head of the Moral Majority organization, with close political ties to the administration of Ronald Reagan, president during the early years of the epidemic. Falwell is also a self-styled biblical scholar, and "Executive Editor" of the *Liberty Bible Commentary* (Nashville, TN: Thomas Nelson, 1983), in which homosexuality is configured as an apocalyptic signifier. In a gloss on Romans 1:26–27, the commentary claims that "Homosexuality is likewise the result of idolatry. . . . Increased homosexuality is a sign of the soon return of the Lord (II Tim 3:2)" (2211). In a reading of the story of the destruction of Sodom and Gomorrah, the editors allude to this passage from the Letter of Paul to the Romans: "Romans reveals that this [homosexuality] is the last stage in a society before it is destroyed" (55).

2. See Anita Bryant's *The Anita Bryant Story: The Survival of Our Nation's Families and the Threat of Militant Homosexuality* (Old Tappan, NJ: Fleming H. Revell Co., 1977), 29–30.

3. Bryant, *Anita Bryant Story*, 42.

4. For a discussion of this prophecy conference and its implications, see Paul Boyer's sixth chapter, "The Final Chastisement of the Chosen," in *When Time Shall Be No More: Prophecy Belief in Modern American Culture* (Cambridge, MA: Belknap/Harvard University Press, 1992). See Harold John Ockenga's "Fulfilled and Unfulfilled Prophecy," in *Prophecy in the Making: Messages Prepared for Jerusalem Conference on Biblical Prophecy*, ed. Carl F. H. Henry (Carol Stream, IL: Creation House, 1971), 291–311; and Wilbur M. Smith's "Signs of the Second Advent of Christ," in *Prophecy in the Making*, 187–213.

5. See David Edwin Harrell's *All Things Are Possible: The Healing and Charismatic Revivals in Modern America* (Bloomington, IN: Indiana University Press, 1975), 186–87; David Wilkerson's *The Vision* (Old Tappan, NJ: Fleming H. Revell Co., 1974), 50–51.

6. See Tim LaHaye's *What Everyone Should Know about Homosexuality*, 4th printing. (Wheaton, IL: Living Books, 1978), especially 8, 11, 203–4. (The book was originally published as *The Unhappy Gays*.) LaHaye is now famous as the coauthor (with Jerry B. Jenkins) of a series of apocalypse novels, the "Left Behind" series, published by Harvest House. Books in the series have regularly appeared on the *New York Times* Best Sellers List and are aggressively marketed in national chain bookstores.

7. See David Chilton, *Power in the Blood: A Christian Response to AIDS* (Brentwood, TN: Wolgemuth & Hyatt, Publishing, 1987), 39; and David Noebel, *The Homosexual Revolution: A Look at the Preachers and Politicians Behind It*, 3rd ed. (Manitou Springs, CO: Summit Press, 1984), 27.

8. William Dannemeyer, *Shadow in the Land: Homosexuality in America* (San Francisco: Ignatius Press, 1989), 222–23.

9. Ed Rowe, *Homosexual Politics: Road to Ruin for America*, intro. Sen. Jesse Helms (Washington, DC: Church League of America, 1984), 12, 24–25, 36.

10. Pierre Bourdieu, *Language and Symbolic Power*, ed. John B. Thompson, trans. Gino Raymond and Matthew Adamson (Cambridge, MA: Harvard University Press, 1991), 40; Robert Hodge, *Literature as Discourse: Textual Strategies in English and History* (Baltimore: Johns Hopkins University Press, 1990), 17.

11. Barry Brumett, *Contemporary Apocalyptic Rhetoric*, Praeger Series in Political Communication, ed. Robert E. Denton, Jr. (New York: Praeger, 1991), 6; M. H. Abrams, "Apocalypse: Theme and Variations," in *The Apocalypse in English Renaissance Thought and Literature*, ed. C. A. Patrides and Joseph Wittreich (Ithaca, NY: Cornell University Press, 1984), 342–68; and Ernest R. Sandeen, *The Roots of Fundamentalism: British and American Millenarism, 1800–1930* (Chicago: University of Chicago Press, 1970). See also Debra Bergoffen, "The Apocalyptic Meaning of History," *The Apocalyptic Vision in America: Interdisciplinary Essays on Myth and Culture*, ed. Lois Parkinson Zamora (Bowling Green, OH: Bowling Green University Popular Press, 1982), 11–36. Henry F. May's *The Enlightenment in America* (New York: Oxford University Press, 1976) proposes a millennialist foundation for late eighteenth-century revolutions. In "Apocalypse: Theme and Variations" M. H. Abrams finds links between apocalypticism and Karl Marx's faith in history, a claim that Ernest L. Tuveson finds supported in the foundational Marxian text ("The Millenarian Structure of *The Communist Manifesto*," ed. Patrides and Wittreich 323–41).

12. Paul Ricoeur, *The Symbolism of Evil*, trans. Emerson Buchanan (Boston: Beacon Press, 1967), 171, 204; Charles H. Lippy, "Waiting for the End: The Social Context of American Apocalyptic Religion," ed. Zamora, 37–63.

13. I. P. Couliano, *Out of This World: Otherworldly Journeys from Gilgamesh to Albert Einstein* (Boston: Shambhala, 1991), 111–12. *Apocalypse of Peter*, ed. and trans. Edgar Hennecke and Wilhelm Schneemelcher, *New Testament Apocrypha*, vol. 2 (Philadelphia: Westminster Press, 1963), 671–81; rep. in *The Other Bible*, ed. Willis Barnstone (San Francisco: HarperSanFrancisco, 1984), 532–36. *Apocalypse of Paul*, ed. and trans. Hennecke and Schneemelcher, 759–60, 764, 773–94, 795, 798; rep. in Barnstone, ed., 537–50.

14. Bernard Capp, "The Political Dimensions of Apocalyptic Thought," Patrides and Wittreich, 93–124; Ricoeur, *Symbolism of Evil*, 28–33.

15. Julia Kristeva, *Powers of Horror: An Essay on Abjection*, trans. Leon S. Roudiez (New York: Columbia University Press, 1982), 4, 53, 205, 207. See also Georges Bataille, *The Accursed Share: An Essay on General Economy*, vol. 2; *The History of Eroticism*, trans. Robert Hurley (New York: Zone, 1991), 95–101; and *Erotism: Death and Sensuality*, trans. Mary Dalwood (San Francisco: City Lights Books, 1986), 107–8.

16. Rist's essay from the *Nation* and some of its replies were reprinted in the New York gay magazine *Christopher Street*, 11, no. 11. Among his respondents were Gore Vidal, Martin Duberman, Jeffrey Escoffier, ACT UP, and Jewelle L. Gomez (11–20).

17. Susan Sontag, *AIDS and Its Metaphors* (New York: Farrar, Straus, Giroux, 1988), especially 78, 88, 93.

18. James Miller, "Dante on Fire Island: Reinventing Heaven in the AIDS Elegy," in *Writing AIDS: Gay Literature, Language, and Analysis*, ed. Timothy Murphy and Suzanne Poirier (New York: Columbia University Press, 1993), 265–305; Michael Lynch, "Terrors of Resurrection 'by Eve Kosofsky Sedgwick,' " in *Confronting AIDS through Literature: The Responsibilities of Representation*, ed. Judith Pastore (Urbana, IL: University of Illinois Press, 1993), 79–83; Peter Dickinson, " 'Go-go Dancing on the Brink of the Apocalypse': Representing AIDS," in *Postmodern Apocalypse: Theory and Cultural Practice at the End*, ed. Richard Dellamora (Philadelphia: University of Pennyslvania Press, 1995), 219–40.

19. Catherine Keller, *Apocalypse Now and Then: A Feminist Guide to the End of the World* (Boston: Beacon Press, 1996), 28; Tina Pippin, *Apocalyptic Bodies: The Biblical End of the World in Text and Image* (New York: Routledge, 1999), 125.

20. Lee Quinby, *Anti-Apocalypse: Exercises in Genealogical Criticism* (Minneapolis, MN: University of Minnesota Press, 1994); *Millennial Seduction: A Skeptic Confronts Apocalyptic Culture* (Ithaca, NY: Cornell University Press, 1999), 41.

21. Richard Dellamora, "Introduction," *Apocalyptic Overtures: Sexual Politics and the Sense of an Ending* (New Brunswick, NJ: Rutgers University Press, 1994), 1–28; Michel Foucault, *The History of Sexuality: An Introduction*, vol. 1, trans. Robert Hurley (New York: Vintage, 1980), 102. See also Dellamora, ed., *Postmodern Apocalypse: Theory and Cultural Practice at the End* (Philadelphia: University of Pennsylvania Press, 1995), especially his introduction (1–14) and "Queer Apocalypse: Framing William Burroughs" (136–70).

22. Bartlett (London: Serpent's Tail, 1988); Hollinghurst (New York: Vintage, 1989).

23. Dellamora, "Afterword" 192–95.

24. I am indebted to three theorists in fashioning this social semiotic praxis. Robert Hodge's *Literature as Discourse: Textual Strategies in English and History* (Baltimore: Johns Hopkins University Press, 1990), first came to my attention in 1991, and confirmed an insight that had been gaining wider currency throughout the 1980s that "English" or "literary studies" were inexorably becoming culture studies and semiotics. Later, I discovered Hodge and Gunther Kress's collaborative *Social Semiotics* (Ithaca, NY: Cornell University Press, 1988), a set of analytical tools applicable to diverse forms of human sign making. Finally, here I refer to Bourdieu's *Language and Symbolic Power*, ed. John B. Thompson, trans. Gino Raymond and Matthew Adamson (Cambridge, MA: Harvard University Press, 1991).

25. Hodge and Kress, *Social Semiotics*, 6.

26. Hodge and Kress, *Social Semiotics*, 3.

27. Hodge, *Literature as Discourse*, 13.

28. Hodge and Kress, *Social Semiotics*, 12.

29. Hodge, *Literature as Discourse*, 13, 21.

30. Hodge, *Literature as Discourse*, 23; Hodge also asserts that the relationship of genre and domain is necessarily complex and he proposes a set of propositions to guide their analysis:

> 1. Genre and domain encode rules that constrain the legitimate production and reception of meaning. . . . They do not present the only meanings of texts. . . . 2. Genre and domain encode rules and knowledges that are important social facts, which must be communicated with massive redundancy if they are to have the force they do, through a large number of metatexts . . . 3. Individual texts typically encode instructions as to how they should be read, and these instructions include prescriptions of genre and domain. (27)

31. Pierre Bourdieu, in *Langauge and Symbolic Power*, a critique of religious and political discourse that builds on J. L. Austin's notion of "performative utterances," observes that the "mystery of performative magic is thus resolved in the mystery of ministry (to use a pun close to the heart of medieval canonists), that is, in the alchemy of *representation* (in the different senses of the term) through which the representative creates the group which creates him" (106). In an analysis of theatrical performance in *Literature as Discourse*, Hodge observes the "meanings that both link and oppose verbal text (script) and performance text (theatrical action)" (58), while he notes that the performance of festivals is a "privileged space for the expression of oppositional meanings" (65).

32. Hodge, *Literature as Discourse*, 88–89.

33. The allegorical typology of apocalyptic narrative is akin to riddling. Hodge notes that:

> The riddle form constructs a doubled text with a doubled modality-value. The individual clauses seem almost nonsense, which has very low modality-value, but the real meaning they conceal has correspondingly high modality, for those that can decode it. The strategy constructs a double community, those who understand/believe and those who are excluded by incomprehension or disbelief. . . . Here . . . the strategy is sustained by attributing great power to the one who alone knows, at some level, the 'sense' of the non-sense, and whose mysteriousness underpins the cohesion and power of the group. (169)

34. Catharine Keller offers a reading of Christopher Columbus' apocalyptic aspirations in her chapter "De/Colon/izing Spaces," in *Apocalypse Now and Then*, 140–80. See also Pauline Moffitt Watts, "Prophesy and Discovery: On the Spiritual Origins of Christopher Columbus' 'Enterprise in the Indies,'" *American Historical Review* 90, no. 1

(February 1985): 73–102. Lois Parkinson Zamora contends that "apocalypse, one of our most basic yet least understood myths, has always been essential to America's conception of itself" and argues that "[f]rom Puritan times onward, much of America's best literature has been apocalyptic, questioning our individual and collective bonds to the world's time and to the world's end" (*Writing the Apocalypse: Historical Vision in Contemporary U.S. and Latin American Fiction* [Cambridge: Cambridge University Press, 1989], 6), and "The Myth of Apocalypse and the American Literary Imagination," ed. Zamora *The Apocalyptic Vision in America: Interdisciplinary Essays on Myth and Culture* (Bowling Green, OH: Bowling Green UniversityPopular Press, 1982), 97–138. Charles H. Lippy argues that American social and political realities have prepared a particularly fertile ground for apocalyptic thought: "Adoption of apocalyptic symbols seemed a logical means to elevate those outside the circles of power to a superior status. . . . The social fluidity of westward expansion, the abolitionist movement and other efforts at social reform, and the unsteady growth of American political institutions all left a feeling of personal and social dislocation among large numbers of Americans who felt excluded from the power, prestige, and security which national leaders seemed to extol" ("Waiting for the End: The Social Context of American Apocalyptic Religion," ed. Zamora, 37–63). While Lippy cites ninteenth-century groups like Shakers, Christadelphians, Millerites, Jehovah's Witnesses, and even Native American Ghost Dancers to illustrate his claim, and cites conservative fundamentalism, with its strong apocalyptic strains, "rebelling against liberal optimism," Ernest R. Sandeen argues that the base of support for early twentieth-century Fundamentalism was urban and middle class, often affluent, though decidedly apocalyptic in its theological origins (*The Roots of Fundamentalism: British and American Millenarism, 1800–1930* [Chicago: University of Chicago Press, 1970]). Sandeen asserts that "it is millenarianism which gave life and shape to the Fundamentalist movement" (xv) and that "Fundamentalism ought to be understood partly if not largely as one aspect of the history of millenarianism" (xix). He also notes that the paradox that persists in modern Fundamentalism was present in early millennialists:

> Their aim was to awaken the sleeping church to the imminence of judgment and to call sinners to repentance before the day of salvation passed away. Although apparently paradoxical, it is possible to show that the millenarians were at the same time convinced of the irreversibly downgrade tendencies at work in human society and the utter futility of attempts to ameliorate the effects of sin, while working for the success of their own movement when that success was defined as awakening Christians to their peril. (xvii)

He also documents tropes of infection which were already a part of Fundamentalist discourse in the early twentieth century: a July 1919 article in *Biblical World*, entitled "The Premillennial Menace" (an attack on Christians who believed that the tribulation before the thousand years of peace had not yet come) condemned those Christians as unpatriotic and defeatist in the war effort and characterized them as a "spiritual virus" (quoted 236). That same year at a conference at which the World's Christian Fundamentals Association was founded, conference organizers condemned the apostasy that was "spreading like a plague throughout Christendom" (quoted. 243). Ernest Tuveson contends that "[w]hen urgent and baffling questions about the right course for the nation have arisen, the apocalyptic view of its history has come to the front: as such times as the expansionist eras, the Civil War, the First World War" (*Redeemer Nation: The Idea of America's Millennial Role* [Chicago: University of Chicago Press, 1968]). Richard Hofstadter finds apocalyptic traces in the propensity toward crisis and conspiracy theories in American politics, what Hoftstadter characterized as "The Paranoid Style," which includes a demonization of threatening minorities (including Catholics, Masons, and Mormons) by fantasizing their sexual excesses and sadism ("The Paranoid Style in American Politics," in *The Fear of Conspiracy: Images of Un-American Subversion from the Revolution to the Present,* ed. David Brion Davis (Ithaca, NY: Cornell University Press, 1971), 2–9; rep. from Richard Hofstadter, *The Paranoid Style in American Politics* (New York: Alfred A. Knopf, 1964, 1965). In the same collection David Brion Davis's "Some Themes of Countersubversion: An Analysis of Anti-Masonic, Anti-Catholic, and Anti-Mormon Literature," documents the rhetoric used against these three groups by dominant Protestant nativists:

> While nativists affirmed their faith in Protestant monogamy, they obviously took pleasure in imagining the variety of sexual experience supposedly available to their enemies. By picturing themselves exposed to similar temptations, they assumed they could know how priests and Mormons actually sinned. . . . We should recall that this literature was written in a period of increasing anxiety and uncertainty over sexual values and the proper role of woman. As ministers and journalists pointed with alarm at the spread of prostitution, the incidence of divorce, and the lax and hypocritical morality of the growing cities, a discussion of licentious subversives offered a convenient means for the projection of guilt as well as desire. The sins of individuals, or of the nation as a whole, could be pushed off upon the shoulders of the enemy and there punished in righteous anger. (18–19)

J. F. Maclear points out in "The Republic and the Millennium," (*The Religion of the Republic,* ed. Elwyn A. Smith [Philadelphia: Fortress, 1971]) that during the second half of the nineteenth century, America's apocalyptic sense of mission "had been readily absorbed by Americans of every creed or none in the increasingly pluralistic post-Civil War society. . . . All could share the inchoate conviction that the Republic constituted a divinely favored nation . . . fulfilling a worthy mission in directing all peoples to democracy, progress, and civilization" (213).

35. Several book-length studies provide useful background for understanding apocalypticism as a pervasive ideology and discourse. Noted earlier, Barry Brummett's *Contemporary Apocalyptic Rhetoric* (Praeger Series in Political Communication, ed. Robert E. Denton, Jr. [New York: Praeger, 1991]) distinguishes three constituencies for millennialist discourse: hard-core religious believers, believers who are less focused, but still persuaded by apocalyptic rhetoric, and the utterly secular (3). Both Stephen D. O'Leary in *Arguing the Apocalypse: A Theory of Millennial Rhetoric* (New York: Oxford University Press, 1994) and Paul Boyer in *When Time Shall Be No More: Prophecy Belief in Modern American Culture* posit the roots of this millennialism in early American antecedents. Robert Fuller draws a similar genealogy while focusing on demonizing in his *Naming the Antichrist: The History of an American Obsession* (New York: Oxford, 1995).

36. See Paul Boyer's *When Time Shall Be No More: Prophecy Belief in Modern American Culture*, 56, 225; Pauline Moffitt Watts's "Prophecy and Discovery: On the Spiritual Origins of Christopher Columbus's 'Enterprise of the Indies,'" *American Historical Review* 90, no. 1 (February 1985): 73–102; Leonard Sweet's "Christopher Columbus and the Millennial Vision of the New World," *Catholic Historical Review* 122 (1986): 369–89; and Djelal Kadir's *Columbus and the Ends of the Earth: Europe's Prophetic Rhetoric as Conquering Ideology* (Berkeley: University of California Press, 1992).

37. As Jonathan Goldberg notes in *Sodometries: Renaissance Texts, Modern Sexualities* (Stanford, CA: Stanford University Press, 1992): "Sodomy is not, as [Alan Bray] sees it, so much a set of forbidden acts as the performance of those undefined acts—or the accusation of their performance—by those who threatened social stability—heretics, spies, traitors, Catholics" (17). At the same time he points out that the definition of *sodomy* is fluid and evasive and will "emerge into visibility only when those are said to have done them also can be called traitors, heretics, or the like, at the very least, disturbers of the social order that alliance—marriage arrangements—maintained" (19).

38. The term "apocalyptic vehemence" is Michael Warner's in "New English Sodom" (*American Literature* 64, no. 1 (March 1992): 19–47) 21, to whose discussion I am indebted. For a study of the frequency of Colonial legal persecution of sodomy, see Robert Oaks, " 'Things Fearful to Name': Sodomy and Buggery in Seventeenth-Century New England" (*The American Man*, ed. Elizabeth and Joseph Pleck [Englewood Cliffs, NJ: Prentice-Hall, 1980], 53–76) where the semantic slippage among "sodomy," "buggery," and "bestiality" is noted.

39. Cassara 69; Tuveson 6–7, 91–174; Kathleen Verduin, " 'Our Cursed Natures': Sexuality and the Puritan Conscience" *The New England Quarterly* 56, no. 2 (June 1983): 220–37.

40. Fuller 68–73; Lakshmi Mani, *The Apocalyptic Vision in Nineteenth Century American Fiction: A Study of Cooper, Hawthorne, and Melville* (Washington, DC: University Press of America, 1981), 43; Henry F. May, *The Enlightenment in America*; J. F. Maclear 183–216. For a further discussion of American literary apocalypses, see Zbigniew Lewicki's *The Bang and the Whimper: Apocalypse and Entropy in American Literature*, Contributions in American Studies, No. 71 (Westport, CT: Greenwood Press, 1984). In her edited collection, Lois Parkinson Zamora's essay, "The Myth of Apocalypse and The American Literary Imagination," is a useful summary of these issues, which she discusses in greater detail in *Writing the Apocalypse: Historical Vision in Contemporary U.S. and Latin American Fiction* (Cambridge: Cambridge University Press, 1989), especially chapter 1, "Introduction: The Apocalyptic Vision and Fictions of Historical Desire." Douglas Robinson covers similar ground in *American Apocalypses: The Image of the End of the World in American Literature* (Baltimore: Johns Hopkins University Press, 1985), as does John R. May's *Toward a New Earth: Apocalypse in the American Novel* (South Bend, IN: University of Notre Dame Press, 1972). David Ketterer focuses on the paraliterary science fiction genre in his *New Worlds for Old: The Apocalyptic Imagination, Science Fiction, and American Literature* (Bloomington, IN: Indiana University Press, 1974).

41. In *The Enlightenment in America*, Henry May observes that, "Philadelphia, especially in the 1790's, was the capital not only of the American Enlightenment, but also

of American culture. For a decade America had a capital which fulfilled, on a small scale, some of the functions of London and Paris" (197). He also points out that, "The gaiety and extravagance of Philadelphia society hardly reached Parisian levels, but nevertheless shocked those natives and visitors who clung to the Spartan principles of Commonwealth ideology" (203).

42. J. H. Powell, *Bring Out Your Dead: The Great Plague of Yellow Fever in Philadelphia in 1793* (Philadelphia: University of Pennsylvania Press, 1949), 283; Norman S. Grabo, "Historical Essay," *Charles Brockden Brown: Arthur Mervyn, or Memoirs of the Year 1793, First and Second Parts,* Bicentennial Edition, ed. Sydney J. Krause (Kent, OH: Kent State University Press, 1980), 447–75.

43. Charles Brockden Brown, *Arthur Mervyn; or, Memoirs of the Year 1793,* ed. Warner Berthoff (New York: Holt, Rinehart, Winston, 1962), 147; hereafter cited in text.

44. Mathew Carey, *A Short Account of the Malignant Fever, Lately Prevalent in Philadelphia,* 4th ed. (Philadelphia, 1794), The Rise of Urban America series, ed. Richard C. Wade (New York: Arno Press, 1970), 10. The *Advertiser* is quoted in John C. Miller, *Crisis in Freedom: The Alien and Sedition Acts* (Boston: Little, Brown, 1951), 40; Alan Axelrod, *Charles Brockden Brown: An American Tale* (Austin, TX: University of Texas Press, 1983), 159; Carey 86–87.

45. The *Gazette* quoted in John C. Miller, *Crisis in Freedom: The Alien and Sedition Acts* (Boston: Little, Brown, 1951), 40; Shirley Samuels, "Infidelity and Contagion: The Rhetoric of Revolution," *Early American Literature* 22 (1987): 183–91; quotes from 183, 188.

46. Shirley Samuels, "Plague and Politics in 1793: *Arthur Mervyn,*" *Criticism* 27, no. 3 (1985): 225–46; quote from 225.

47. I am paying particular attention to the historical or material conditions of the production of meaning among gay men and others in New York City. In doing so, I have found several studies useful in understanding the social background. Steven Seidman's *Romantic Longings: Love in America, 1830–1980* (New York: Routledge, 1991) and John D'Emilio and Estelle B. Freedman's *Intimate Matters: A History of Sexuality in America* (New York: Harper & Row, 1988) both document the varieties of sexuality in different American communities across time. George Chauncey's *Gay New York: Gender, Urban Culture, and the Making of the Gay Male World 1890–1940* (New York: BasicBooks, 1994) is a remarkable demythologizing of urban America's queer past that establishes the grounds for New York's iconic role in modern gay life. A good general history of gay and lesbian lives can be found Neil Miller's in *Out of the Past: Gay and Lesbian History from 1869 to the Present* (New York: Vintage Books, 1995); it relates an accessible narrative of the Christian fundamentalist antigay backlash of the 1970s and the onset of AIDS in the 1980s. Focusing on the period between the end of World War II and Stonewall, John D'Emilio documents lesbian and gay visibility and activism in his *Sexual Politics, Sexual Communities: The Making of a Homosexual Minority in the United States, 1940–1970* (Chicago: University of Chicago Press, 1983). Historian Martin Duberman presents the most detailed account of modern gay activism, much of it occurring in New York City, in his *Stonewall* (New York: Plume, 1993). Martin P. Levine's "The Life and Death of Gay Clones" (*Gay Culture in America: Essays from the Field,* ed. Gilbert Herdt [Boston: Beacon Press, 1992], 68–86) provides a sociological study of New York's most visibly

AIDS affected, gay men living in lower Manhattan in or around Greenwich Village and Chelsea in the 1970s and 1980s. Stephen O. Murray's more recent *American Gay* (Chicago: University of Chicago Press, 1996) offers a social analysis of homosexual identity across race lines in North America.

Notes to Chapter Two

1. See William L. Leap's fifth chapter, "Claiming Gay Space: Bathroom Graffiti, Songs about Cities, and 'Queer' Reference," in his *Word's Out: Gay Men's English* (Minneapolis, MN: University of Minnesota Press, 1996) for a discussion of the exile trope in gay men's popular culture. In his "psychohistory," *The Stonewall Experiment* (London: Cassell, 1995), Ian Young offers a mythological reading of *The Wizard of Oz*. Reminding us that U.S. concerns are often provincial, Simon Watney discusses the international implications of identity politics in "AIDS and the Politics of Queer Diaspora," in *Negotiating Lesbian and Gay Subjects*, ed. Monica Dorenkamp and Richard Henke (New York: Routledge, 1995), 53–70.

2. James McCourt, *Time Remaining* (New York: Alfred A. Knopf, 1993); Tim Miller, "My Queer Body" *Sharing the Delirium: Second Generation AIDS Plays and Performances*, ed. Therese Jones (Portsmouth, NH: Heinemann, 1994), 309–36; David Drake, *The Night Larry Kramer Kissed Me*, foreword by Michelangelo Signorile (New York: Anchor Books, 1992). Hereafter all cited in the text.

3. Stephen D. O'Leary, *Arguing the Apocalypse: A Theory of Millennial Rhetoric* (New York: Oxford University Press, 1994), 200–206.

4. Jody Berland, "Angels Dancing: Cultural Technologies and the Production of Space," in *Cultural Studies*, ed. Lawrence Grossberg, Cary Nelson, and Paula Treichler (New York: Routledge, 1992), 38–55; quote from 39; "The HIV/AIDS Epidemic in New York City," *The Social Impact of AIDS in the United States*, ed. Albert R. Jonsen and Jeff Stryker, Report of the Committee on AIDS Research and Behavioral, Social, and Statistical Sciences, National Research Council (Washington, DC: National Academy Press, 1993), 244–45.

5. George Chauncey, *Gay New York: Gender, Urban Culture, and the Making of the Gay Male World 1890–1940* (New York: BasicBooks, 1994), 1–29. See also Eric Garber's "A Spectacle in Color: The Lesbian and Gay Subculture of Jazz Age Harlem," in *Hidden from History: Reclaiming the Gay and Lesbian Past*, ed. Martin Duberman, Martha Vicinus, and George Chauncey (New York: Meridian Books, 1989), 318–31. Allen Bérubé offers a ground breaking account of gays in World War II in *Coming Out Under Fire: Lesbian and Gay Americans and the Military During World War II* (New York: Free Press, 1989). For a related discussion, see John D'Emilio's second chapter, "Forging a Group Identity: World War II and the Emergence of an Urban Gay Subculture," in his *Sexual Politics, Sexual Communities: The Making of a Homosexual Minority in the United States, 1940–1970* (Chicago: University of Chicago Press, 1983). A new theoretical awareness of the relationship between physical spaces and sexuality is evident in two critical collections: Gordon Brent Ingram, Anne-Marie Bouthillette, and Yolanda Retter, eds., *Queers in*

Space: Communities, Public Places, Sites of Resistance (Seattle: Bay Press, 1997) and David Bell and Gill Valentine, eds., *Mapping Desire: Geographies of Sexualities* (New York: Routledge, 1995), both of which assemble diverse microanalyses and local histories. For a more theoretically unified treatment, see Daphne Spain's *Gendered Spaces* (Chapel Hill, NC: University of North Carolina Press, 1992).

6. *The Gay Insider: A Hunter's Guide to New York and a Thesaurus of Phallic Lore* (New York: Traveller's Companion, 1971).

7. Jonsen and Stryker, *Social Impact of AIDS*, 295.

8. Richard Schechner, *Between Theater and Anthropology*, foreword by Victor Turner, (Philadelphia: University of Pennsylvania Press, 1985), 79.

9. Performer and writer Holly Hughes joined academic culture critic David Román in editing a collection of thirteen solo-performance "scripts" in *O Solo Homo: The New Queer Performance* (New York: Grove Press, 1998), including a coauthored introduction, Tim Miller's *Naked Breath*, Ron Vawter's *Roy Cohn/Jack Smith*, and Hughes's own *Clit Notes*.

10. The text of the Abdohs' *Quotations from a Ruined City* can be found in *The Drama Review* 39, no. 4 (Fall 1995): 108–36. The same issue includes several articles on and interviews with the late Reza Abdoh.

11. Judith Butler, "Imitation and Gender Insubordination," *Inside/Out: Lesbian Theories, Gay Theories*, ed. Diana Fuss (New York: Routledge, 1991), 13–31; *Gender Trouble: Feminism and the Subversion of Identity* (New York: Routledge, 1990); "Queer Performativity: Henry James's *The Art of the Novel*," *GLQ* 1, no. 1 (1993): 1–16; quotes from 11, 14. Butler and Sedgwick have subsequently offered refinements to their earlier work, Butler in *Bodies That Matter: On the Discursive Limits of "Sex"* (New York: Routledge, 1993) and Sedgwick in *Tendencies* (Durham, NC: Duke University Press, 1993).

12. Butler, "Critically Queer" *GLQ* 1, no. 1 (1993): 17–32; quote from 28; Peggy Phelan, *Unmarked: The Politics of Performance* (New York: Routledge, 1993) 101; David Román, "It's My Party and I'll Die If I Want To!: Gay Men, AIDS, and the Circulation of Camp in U.S. Theater," in *Camp Grounds: Style and Homosexuality*, ed. David Bergman (Amherst: University Mass Press, 1993), 206–33; quote from 220.

13. Cohen, "Who Are 'We'? Gay 'Identity' as Political (E)motion (A Theoretical Rumination)" Fuss 71–92; quote from 89.

14. Pierre Bourdieu, *Language and Symbolic Power*, ed. John B. Thompson, trans. Gino Raymond and Matthew Adamson (Cambridge. MA: Harvard University Press, 1991), 40.

15. David Román, 218; Jill Dolan, "Practicing Cultural Disruptions: Gay and Lesbian Representation and Sexuality," in *Critical Theory and Performance*, ed. Janelle G. Reinelt and Joseph R. Roach (Ann Arbor: University of Michigan Press, 1992), 263–75, quote from 272; Robert Wallace, "Performance Anxiety: 'Identity,' 'Community,' and Tim Miller's My Queer Body," *Modern Drama* 39 (1996): 97–116; Marvin Carlson, *Performance: A Critical Introduction* (London: Routledge, 1996), 173, 174; Phelan 10–11. Almost from the beginning of the AIDS epidemic, culture workers in academia and in the arts have struggled with the question of how productive their efforts are in the midst

of death. A classic articulation of the problem is Douglas Crimp's "AIDS: Cultural Analysis/Cultural Activism," (from the book he edited, *AIDS: Cultural Analysis/Cultural Activism* [Cambridge, MA: MIT Press, 1987], 3–16), which suggests that artists can produce both information and mobilization. In "The Spectacle of AIDS," Simon Watney asserts that cultural critics play an important role in undermining uncritical representations of AIDS (Crimp, *Cultural Analysis,* 71–86).

16. Burt Supree, "Jerk Off for Jesse," *Village Voice,* January 7, 1992; Robin Dougherty, "Body/double: Miller's Tale at the Charles," *Boston Phoenix,* October 9, 1992; Kevin Thaddeus Paulson, "Blood, Breath, Death and Sex," San Francisco *Sentinel,* May 4, 1994; Anne Marie Welsh, "Miller can be wonderful to unQueer Nation, too," San Diego *Union-Tribune* January 17, 1995.

17. Malcolm Boyd and Nancy L. Wilson, eds. *Amazing Grace: Stories of Lesbian and Gay Faith* (Freedom, CA: Crossing Press, n.d.), 57–66.

18. I interviewed Miller on August 10, 1995. See also Jeff Weinstein, review of Tim Miller's *Naked Breath, Village Voice,* December 13, 1994, 104; Robert Nesti, "Lust at First Sight," *Bay Windows,* September 22, 1994, 21; Tim Miller and David Román, "Preaching to the Converted," *Theatre Journal* 47 (1995): 169–88; Lizbeth Goodman, "Bodies and Stages: An Interview with Tim Miller," *Critical Quarterly* 36, no. 1 (Spring 1994): 63–72; Jan Breslauer, "Art = Activism," *Los Angeles Times Magazine* December 1, 1991; Misha Berson, "For Tim Miller, A Stripped-Down Performance," *Seattle Times,* May 12, 1993; and Steven Durland, "An Anarchic, Subversive, Erotic Soul: An Interview with Tim Miller," *Drama Review* 35, no. 3 (Fall 1991): 171–77.

19. Miller and Román, "Preaching," 177–78, 178–79, 186.

20. Miller and Román, "Preaching," 188.

21. As Peggy Phelan observes in her critique of the film, *Paris is Burning,* whose subject is the drag culture of black and Latino gay men in New York:

> The extravagant costume and *personae* displayed at the balls are serious rehearsals for a much tougher walk—down the "mean streets" of New York City. The balls are opportunities to use theatre to imitate the theatricality of everyday life—a life which includes show girls, bangee boys, and business executives. It is the endless theatre of everyday life that determines the real: and this theatricality is soaked through with racial, sexual, and class bias. (98–99)

See Holleran's "Ground Zero" in *Ground Zero,* 28.

22. The "NEA Four" also included John Fleck, Karen Finley, and Holly Hughes. For a discussion of the NEA funding controversy and its effects on the artists, see William Harris's "The N.E.A. Four: Life after Symbolhood," *New York Times,* June 5, 1994, section 2, 1; and C. Reid and M. O'Brien's "Court rejection of NEA 'decency standard' viewed as 'breakthrough,' " *Publishers Weekly,* June 15, 1992, 8–9. For a more detailed analysis, see Steven C. Dubin's *Arresting Images: Impolitic Art and Uncivil Actions* (New York: Routledge, 1992).

23. Jack Anderson, "Portraits of Gay Men, with No Apologies," *New York Times* January 10, 1993. See also Lizbeth Goodman, "Bodies and Stages," 71–72; and Berson.

24. Peggy Phelan observes that "The desire to see is a manifestation of the desire to be seen, in live performance as well as in the spectator's relation to inanimate representation. All vision doubts and hopes for a response" (18). Live performance deploys identities in ways that reproductions cannot in that "the exchange of gaze marks the split *within* the subject (the loss of the Specular I of the Imaginary) and *between* subjects (the entry into the Social I of the Symbolic). The 'here/there' articulated with Lacan's story of the sardine can, and also elaborated in his commentary on Freud's *fort/da* game, reflects the linguistic distinction between the positions of 'I' and 'it' " (Phelan, 21).

25. See Berson; Breslauer 6; Durland 172–73; Jim Provenzano, "Miller's Crossing," *Bay Area Reporter*, Arts and Entertainment, April 28, 1994.

26. "Death and Dancing in the Live Arts: Performance, Politics and Sexuality in the Age of AIDS," *Critical Quarterly* 35, no. 2 (1993): 99–116; quote on 104.

27. Goodman, "Bodies and Stages," 67–71.

28. Miller Interview. Robert Hodge and Gunther Kress observe that some spaces are designated for rituals of reversal, for those sanctioned periods of carnival when the Freudian repressed is permitted to return (73–78). In an analysis of ancient English festivals, which were forbidden after the Reformation and prosecuted by the Puritans, Hodge observes,

> But festivals did not survive out of attachment to history. They survived because they continued to do semiosic work, serving crucial social functions for small communities. Semiosically, they constituted a privileged space for the expression of oppositional meanings, "midsummer madness," a time of license and inversion of hierarchy and constraint. Their mimetic content was a specific conflation of love (celebration, fecundity, abundance) and death (sacrifice, loss and mourning) in a single package with a double meaning and purpose. The image of death followed by love, growth and regeneration was an equally potent "natural" consolation in time of loss and bereavement. (65)

This kind of ancient human ritual performance took on particular poignancy in the first decade of the AIDS crisis.

29. Sylvie Drake, " 'Night Kramer Kissed Me' a Compelling, Fresh Show," *Los Angeles Times* May 24, 1993: F3. On the poster for *The Night Larry Kramer Kissed Me* fashion and former *Interview* fashion photographer Christopher Makos presented Drake in jeans, shirtless with a leather jacket slipping off his shoulders, an androgynous blending of stereotypical male and female sexuality. During most of the performance, Drake wore tight 501 button-fly jeans with the fabric worn where his penis and scrotum had been tucked in one leg, a signifier of sexual availability.

30. In his review of the play ("Normal Kisses," *Village Voice*, July 7, 1992, Michael Feingold observed that "Drake's intention is to turn his life into a gay myth, an exemplar for generations to come. . . . How well he succeeds depends less on what you think of the life he describes than on how much you value the myth."

31. See Marjorie Kaufman "Stepping Into the Role of 'Gay Everyman,' " *New York Times*, March 14, 1993: LI11; and Alisa Solomon, "The Performance Art That Dare Not Speak Its Name," *Village Voice*, September 29, 1992: 104.

32. "Rash Impulses," review of David Drake's *The Night Larry Kramer Kissed Me* and Josh Kornbluth's *Red Diaper Baby, Time*, July 13, 1992. As with the "Short Takes" double review in *Time* magazine, David Richards ("The Minefields in Monologues," *New York Times*, July 12, 1992), compared Drake's play to Josh Kornbluth's *Red Diaper Baby*, another autobiographical work for solo performer.

33. Richard Dellamora, *Apocalyptic Overtures: Sexual Politics and the Sense of an Ending* (New Brunswick, NJ: Rutgers University Press, 1994), 192. Dellamora composed that comment in an "Afterword" to a book whose final manuscript he had sent to the publisher the day he saw Drake's performance, four days before Drake would leave to perform the role on the West Coast, to be replaced in New York by Eric Paeper.

34. Phelan, *Unmarked*, 146; 150; 178.

35. Miller has objected to Solomon's criticism by saying, "The *Voice* ran this huge article once comparing us and being mean to David. I like his work; his piece is powerful and important work. David's arrival with that work is a strong presence. It's a play, which is different. I want my body to be present in the incarnation of the text" (Interview). The following material summarizes Solomon's critique.

36. Peggy Phelan, "Tim Miller's *My Queer Body*: An Anatomy in Six Sections," *Theater* 24, no. 2 (1993): 30–34.

37. Carlson, *Performance*, 186; Schechner, *Between*, 36

38. Phelan, *Unmarked*, 148, 149; Hodge, *Literature as Discourse*, 58.

39. Pearl K. Bell, "Fiction Chronicle," *Partisan Review* 61 (Winter 1994): 80–95; Wayne Koestenbaum, *The Queen's Throat: Opera, Homosexuality, and the Mystery of Desire* (New York: Poseidon, 1993), 17; Bertha Harris, "In a pink sequined straightjacket," *New York Times*, June 3, 1993. In her review, Pearl K. Bell admitted that *Time Remaining* "is not a novel, though who knows what the right word might be for such an uncorseted, unstoppable romp through the pre-AIDS years of camp culture" (92). The book's form found Walter Kendrick ("Fiction in Review," *Yale Review* 81, no. 4 (1993): 124–37) similarly at an uncharacteristic loss for words: "actually a novel in disguise, or something unnameable disguised as a novel" (126). Sybil Steinberg, review of *Time Remaining, Publishers Weekly*, March 29, 1993: 37 claimed the two parts of the book as novellas. McCourt himself repudiates the category of novel: " 'I don't write novels. . . . The novel is an English middle-class product. It is undeniably wonderful—love Dickens—with plots and all that. Myself, I write tales. They go on and on, then just stop. I belong to the Irish tradition of storytelling. Or as they used to say at the [notorious Manhattan disco] Danceteria: "F——art, let's dance" ' " (quoted in William Hoffman, "The Interior Landscape of James McCourt," *Los Angeles Times Magazine*, October 31, 1995: 30–34; quote from 34).

40. *Mawrdew Czgowchwz* (New York: Farrar, Straus and Giroux, 1975); *Kaye Wayfaring in "Avenged"* (New York: Alfred A. Knopf, 1984); *Delancey's Way* (New York: Knopf, 2000).

41. William Hoffman notes that "McCourt's densely packed prose, like James Joyce's, unlike much contemporary avant-garde fiction, actually *means* something" (30). Anne C. Fullam's interview with McCourt ("A Joycean-Style Memorial to the Dead," *New York Times*, September 12, 1993: LI 21.) characterizes the book as a "prose poem in Joycean style." McCourt quoted in Hoffman 34.

42. Phelan, *Unmarked,* 97.

43. See William L. Leap for a careful discourse analysis of the ways (white, middle-class) gay men use language, particularly in playful forms of competition (*Word's Out: Gay Men's English* [Minneapolis, MN: University of Minnesota Press, 1996]). Performing a similar service for black gay men are two essays in Essex Hemphill's collection, *Brother to Brother* (Boston: Alyson Publications, 1991): Charles I. Nero's "Toward a Black Gay Aesthetic: Signifying in Contemporary Black Gay Literature" (229–52), and Marlon Riggs' "Black Macho Revisited: Reflections of a SNAP! Queen" (253–57).

44. Román, " 'It's My Party,' " 215.

45. Román, " 'It's My Party,' " 219–20.

46. According to Hodge and Kress,

> The motor of semiotic change is the desire to express difference. This desire proceeds from the need of specific groups to create internal solidarity and to exclude others, as antigroups constructing antilanguages, antimeanings, anticultures and antiworlds. . . . Differences can be expressed by marked choices and significant transformations a any level in a semiotic hierarchy, from the micro level ("accent," "style" or "grammar") through the meso level (item, phrase, ensemble) to the macro level (topic, theme, cosmology, metaphysics). . . . These differences exist to express group ideology and group identity. They normally form functional sets of metasigns (pervasive markers of group allegiance), whose meaning is social rather than referential, oriented to the semiosic rather than the mimetic plane. (90)

Gianni Vattimo, *The Transparent Society* (Baltimore: Johns Hopkins University Press, 1992) makes a similar point when he asserts the connection between aesthetics and collective identity:

> If . . . art in the traditional sense of the work of art reverts to order . . . , the site of aesthetic experience in society is shifting: not simply towards the generalization of design and a universal social hygiene with regard to forms, nor even as a Marcusian aesthetico-revolutionary rehabilitation of existence, but rather in the sense of an unfolding of the capacity of the aesthetic product—nowise the work of art—to 'make a world,' to create community. . . . The experience of the beautiful, then, more fundamentally than the experience of a structure we simply find pleasing (yet on the basis of what criteria?), is the experience of belonging to a community. (66, 67)

47. Eve Kosofsky Sedgwick's *Epistemology of the Closet* (Berkeley: University of California Press, 1990) is a central text in the development of "Queer Theory," while the essays collected by Edward Stein in *Forms of Desire: Sexual Orientation and the Social Constructionist Controversy* (New York: Routledge, 1990) articulate several positions in this discussion. Stein's own "Conclusion: The Essentials of Constructionism and the Construction of Essentialism" (325–53) performs a valuable service by problematizing the binary terms of the debate. In many respects, the style of McCourt's writing is camp, defined by Susan Sontag's classic 1964 essay, "Notes on Camp," as "homosexual aestheticism and irony" (118). In *Making Things Perfectly Queer: Interpreting Mass Culture* (Minneapolis, MN: University of Minnesota Press, 1993), Alexander Doty critiques the queerness of popular culture by exploring "queer" as a term that is "more than just an umbrella term in the ways that 'homosexual' and 'gay' have been used to mean lesbian *or* gay *or* bisexual, because queerness can also be about the intersecting or combining of more than one specific form of nonstraight sexuality" (xvi).

48. Kendrick, "Fiction," 128–29.

49. Quoted in Anne C. Fullam, "A Joycean-Style Memorial to the Dead," *New York Times*, September 12, 1993.

50. Roland Barthes, "Theory of the Text," trans. Ian McLeod, *Untying the Text: A Post-Structuralist Reader*, ed. Robert Young (Boston: Routledge & Kegan Paul, 1981), 31–47; quote from 32.

51. Barthes, 39.

52. Barthes, 36, 37.

53. Miller and Román, 177.

54. Leon Festinger, Henry W. Riecken, and Stanley Schachter, *When Prophecy Fails: A Social and Psychological Study of a Modern Group that Predicted the Destruction of the World* (New York: Harper & Row, 1956).

55. Sacvan Bercovitch, *The Puritan Origins of the American Self* (New Haven: Yale University Press, 1975), 24, 136, 144, 186; Carlson 116.

NOTES TO CHAPTER THREE

1. Kramer has twice collected his AIDS-related essays, articles, letters, and speeches in *Reports from the Holocaust: The Story of an AIDS Activist*, first in 1988, and in a revised and expanded edition in 1994 (New York: St. Martin's Press). Because of the book's wide availability, I will cite it whenever possible. See *Reports* 33; Sacvan Bercovitch, *American Jeremiad* (Madison, WI: University of Wisconsin Press, 1978), xi.

2. Bercovitch, *American Jeremiad*, 4.

3. The distinction between prophetic utterance and apocalyptic utterance is not only a product of form (genre) criticism but also of an argument about the origins of apocalypticism, some biblical scholars tracing its origins to Jewish prophetic literature,

others to Mesopotamian and Persian literature. See John J. Collins, *The Apocalyptic Imagination: An Introduction to the Jewish Matrix of Christianity* (New York: Crossroad, 1984) for a full treatment of this issue.

4. Bercovitch, *American Jeremiad,* 10, 23.

5. Bercovitch, *American Jeremiad,* 23.

6. James Miller, "Criticism as Activism," in *Fluid Fluid Exchanges: Artists and Critics in the AIDS Crisis,* ed. James Miller (Toronto: University of Toronto Press, 1992), 185–214; quotation from 196–97; John Nguyet Erni, *Unstable Frontiers: Technomedicine and the Cultural Politics of "Curing" AIDS* (Minneapolis, MN: University of Minnesota Press, 1994), 94.

7. A useful social study of New York's clone culture can be found in Martin P. Levine's "The Life and Death of Gay Clones," in *Gay Culture in America: Essays from the Field,* ed. Gilbert Herdt (Boston: Beacon Press, 1992), 68–86. Two well known fictional accounts of this time and place are Andrew Holleran's *Dancer from the Dance* (New York: William Morrow, 1978) and Edmund White's *Forgetting Elena* (New York: Random House, 1973). An interesting exploration of Seventies disco and today's retro-disco as a trope can be found in a recently published article by Gregory Bredbeck, "Troping the Light Fantastic: Representing Disco Then and Now," *GLQ* 3, no. 1 (1996): 71–107.

8. Kramer, *Reports,* xxxii.

9. *Reports* 6; 4. Since my purpose here is not to adjudicate the "truth" of Kramer's claims or those of his critics, it is enough for me to note that Kramer's earliest critique has shaped his sense of possibility and disappointment throughout his career as an AIDS activist. There can also be little purpose in contesting that gays in San Francisco came to enjoy civil rights years before those were legislated on behalf of gay New Yorkers, and that state and municipal funding for AIDS in San Francisco far exceeded that in New York in the early years of the epidemic, suggesting a disparity in the effectiveness of gay politics in those two cities.

10. James Miller, "Dante on Fire Island: Reinventing Heaven in the AIDS Elegy," in *Writing AIDS: Gay Literature, Language, and Analysis,* ed. Timothy F. Murphy and Suzanne Poirier (New York: Columbia University Press, 1993), 265–305; quote on 270; David Bergman, "Larry Kramer and the Rhetoric of AIDS," in *Gaiety Transfigured: Gay Self-Representation in American Literature* (Madison, WI: University of Wisconsin Press, 1991), 122–38; see 128; Barbara Harrison "Love on the Seedy Side," *Washington Post Book World,* December 17, 1978; Martin Duberman, review of Larry Kramer's *Faggots, New Republic,* January 6, 1979, 30–32.

11. *Faggots* (New York: Random House, 1978), 7; hereafter cited in the text.

12. Randy Shilts in his contested novelistic history of the AIDS epidemic, *And the Band Played On: Politics, People and the AIDS Epidemic* (New York: St. Martin's Press, 1987), discusses these public health concerns of the late 1970s in his second chapter, "Glory Days." Much to Shilts's credit, he had researched and reported earlier in the 70s on the high rates of sexually transmitted diseases among urban gay men, as well as the few government resources ($160,000 out of $33 million for STD treatment) designated for this epidemic (see Shilts, "VD," *Advocate,* April 21, 1976, 14). The late Michael

Callen, New York entertainer, activist, and long-term AIDS survivor recalled these health concerns in his own life and community in the introduction to his *Surviving AIDS* (New York: HarperCollins, 1990).

13. Dr. Lawrence Mass's first article appeared in the same periodical ("Disease Rumors Largely Unfounded," *New York Native*, May 18–31, 1981, 7), and two months after Lawrence Altman's was published in the *Times*, "Rare Cancer Seen in 41 Homosexuals," July 3, 1981, 20; *Reports* 9.

14. *Reports*, 8; Robert Chesley, letter to the editor, *New York Native*, October 18, 1981, 4.

15. *Reports*, 11.

16. *Reports*, 16, 20, 21, 22.

17. Arthur Bell, October 19–November 1, 1981, 4; Nathan Fain, October 19–November, 1, 1981, 4; Scott Tucker, 19 October–1 November, 1981, 4; Tucker would later be strongly critical of Kramer's rhetorical excesses; see *Fighting Words: An Open Letter to Queers and Radicals* (London: Cassell, 1995), especially 46–48.

18. Robert Chesley, Letter, January 4–17, 1982; Owen Wilson, January 4–17, 1982; Francis Xavier Boynton, Jr., Letter, January 4–17, 1982 . "Boynton" was probably George Whitmore, a journalist and fiction writer whose serialized fiction, *Deep Dish* had been appearing in the *Native*. His character, Francis X. Boynton, Jr., was the narrator of the *Deep Dish* tales. "Dish," of course, is camp lingo for "dirt" or "gossip." Ironically, during some of the autumn 1981 installments, the narrator described a character's invitation to a hospital-themed orgy ("CATHERIZATION, EXPLORATORY SURGERY, ACUPUNC-TURE"), whose tag line was, "Are you sick enough to attend?" (Episode 20: "Fleurs du Mal" *New York Native*, September 7–20, 1981, 30).

19. Letter to the Editor, *New York Native*, January 4–17, 1982, 5.

20. Richard Umans, January 18–31, 1982, 4; Arnie Kantrowitz, January 18–31, 1982, 4; Richard Haber, January 18–31, 1982, 4.

21. Michael Hirsch, February 1–14, 1982, 4; Edward Sherman, February 1–14, 1982, 4; Robert Cromwell, February 15–28, 1982, 4; Pete Wilson, February 1–14, 1982, 4.

22. *Reports*, 218–19.

23. *Reports*, 102; 134.

24. *Reports*, 300; "A Few Personal Words," *Newspaper of ACT UP*, September–October, 1989, 2; *Reports* 326, 327. In a letter to the editor accompanying Larry Kramer's February 16, 1987 "open letter" to Tim Sweeney, Vito Russo supported Kramer's charges about GMHC: "Yet the issues raised by Kramer are so real, so vital, and so urgent as to command our consideration . . . yes, attacking GMHC is like spitting on God. What I didn't expect was that GMHC would respond to Kramer as though they really were God" (8). See also *Reports*, 383. Dr. Suzanne Phillips, letter to the editor, *New York Native*, May 7, 1990, 6.

25. *Reports*, 156; 170; 182–83.

26. *Reports,* 193; 197; 198.

27. Arendt, *Eichmann in Jerusalem: A Report on the Banality of Evil,* rev. ed. (New York: Penguin, 1978); *Reports,* 267; 270.

28. *Reports,* 289; 302.

29. *Destiny of Me* (New York: Plume, 1993), hereafter cited in the text; Interview by Beowulf Thorne, *Diseased Pariah News,* No. 9, 1994, 25–30; *Reports,* 417, 419.

30. Pierre Bourdieu, *Language and Symbolic Power,* ed. John B. Thompson; trans. Gino Raymond and Matthew Adamson (Cambridge, MA: Harvard University Press, 1991), 37, 81–89.

31. *The Normal Heart* (New York: Plume, 1985), hereafter cited in the text. Among the documentation printed on the set's panels were the current number of AIDS cases ". . . and counting"; a comparison of the number of times the *New York Times* had published AIDS reports compared to the track record of other metropolitan papers in the United States; statistics comparing New York Mayor Ed Koch's funding for AIDS compared to that of San Francisco's Dianne Feinstein; and so forth, prominently displayed.

32. *Just Say No: A Play about a Farce* (New York: St. Martin's Press, 1989), hereafter cited in the text.

33. *Just Say No,* "Introduction," xxiii.

34. *Reports,* 288; "Why I Think Ed Koch is a Pig," *Outweek,* September 11, 1989, 38–39; *Reports,* 288, 413.

35. *Reports,* 178, 180.

36. Keith Alcorn's "AIDS in the Public Sphere: How a Broadcasting System in Crisis Dealt with an Epidemic" in *Taking Liberties: AIDS and Cultural Politics,* ed. Erica Carter and Simon Watney (London: Serpent's Tail, 1989), 193–212, offers an account of the British media's construction of the AIDS crisis. AIDS did not become a "crisis" for heterosexuals until they began to see their own interests at stake. This began to occur, ironically, with the revelation of closeted homosexual Rock Hudson's AIDS diagnosis in July 1985. That month the *Life* magazine cover announced: "Now No One Is Safe from AIDS." Three years later, William Masters, Virginia Johnson (famed sexologists), and Robert Kolodny would market a seriously flawed and misleading study under the title, *Crisis: Heterosexual Behavior in the Age of AIDS* (New York: Grove Press, 1988), which was featured as the cover story in the March 14, 1988 *Newsweek,* the first time that a cover ever focused on a book. See James Kinsella's *Covering the Plague: AIDS and the American Media* (New Brunswick, NJ: Rutgers University Press, 1989) for a study of the relationship between the epidemic and the mass media.

37. See Neil Miller's Chapter 24, "The 1970s: The Times of Harvey Milk and Anita Bryant," in *Out of the Past: Gay and Lesbian History from 1869 to the Present* (New York: Vintage Books, 1995) for a survey of gay and lesbian activism during this period. Rodger Streitmatter details gay journalism at the same time in "Fighting Back against the New Right" in his *Unspeakable: The Rise of the Gay and Lesbian Press in America* (Boston: Faber and Faber, 1995), 211–42.

38. *New York Native*, February 28–March 13, 1983, 2.

39. *Reports*, 25; 33.

40. The groundbreaking historical research on European society's legal, religious, and cultural responses to homosexuality can be found in John Boswell's *Christianity, Social Tolerance, and Homosexuality: Gay People in Western Europe from the Beginning of the Christian Era to the Fourteenth Century* (Chicago: University of Chicago Press, 1980); Alan Bray's *Homosexuality in Renaissance England* (London: Gay Men's Press, 1982); and Heinz Heger's *The Men with the Pink Triangle* trans. David Fernbach (Boston: Alyson Publications, 1980), a firsthand account of Nazi treatment of gays. For a broader histori- cal view, see Louis Crompton's "Gay Genocide from Leviticus to Hitler," in *The Gay Academic*, ed. Louie Crew (Palm Springs: ETC Publications, 1978), 67–91. John Francis Hunter, *The Gay Insider: A Hunter's Guide to New York and a Thesaurus of Phallic Lore* (New York: The Traveller's Companion, 1971), 73; Alabama Birdstone, *Queer Free* (New York: Calamus Books, 1981); Tim Barrus, *Genocide: The Anthology* (Stamford, CT: Knights Press, 1988).

41. *Reports*, 45–46.

42. Ralph Sepulveda, Jr., *New York Native*, March 28–April 10, 1983, 4–6; Jim Levin, 6; Christopher Lynn, 7; Jurg Mahner, 5. Compare those responses with other critiques of AIDS apocalypticism, particularly the trope of genocide, such as gay conser- vative Bruce Bawer's "Apocalypse? No," in *Beyond Queer: Challenging Gay Left Orthodoxy* (New York: Free Press, 1996, 102–4) and Darrell Yates Rist's controversial "AIDS as Apocalypse: The Deadly Costs of an Obsession," *Nation*, February 13, 1989, 181+. In *Unstable Frontiers: Technomedicine and the Cultural Politics of "Curing" AIDS* (Minneapo- lis, MN: University of Minnesota Press, 1994), John Nguyet Erni argued that much of the dominant discourse on AIDS ("that AIDS is 'invariably fatal,' that HIV is perma- nently monstrous, that all people with AIDS are the clinical embodiment of grotesque disfigurement (of both body and character), that AIDS statistics authorize the de facto sign of inevitable massive deaths") represents what he calls a "fantasy of menace and morbidity" which "seems vindictively eager to imagine a historical prospect of the eradi- cation of 'homosexual acts,' whether carried out by homosexuals or not, and, by exten- sion, the eradication of the figure of the homosexual" (49).

43. *Reports*, 66; *The Normal Heart*, 21–22.

44. Paula Treichler summarizes some of the conspiracy speculations about AIDS in "AIDS, Homophobia, and Biomedical Discourse: An Epidemic of Signification," in *AIDS: Cultural Analysis, Cultural Activism*, ed. Douglas Crimp (Cambridge. MA: MIT Press, 1987), 31–70. James Kinsella notes that New York's Harlem-based *Amsterdam News* spent considerable energy tracking down conspiracy theories about AIDS (*Covering the Plague*, 245). Naming and describing several conspiratorial theories, Dennis Altman concluded in 1986, "I frankly doubt any of these explanations, but one cannot totally dismiss their plausibility;" see *AIDS in the Mind of America* (New York: Doubleday, 1986), 44. Some conspiracy accounts may have been composed abroad, including the Soviet Union where AIDS was perceived as a fascist menace, according to Mirko Grmek in *History of AIDS: Emergence of a Modern Pandemic*, trans. Russell C. Maulitz and Jacalyn Duffin (Princeton:

Princeton University Press, 1990), 151–52. Arthur Frederick Ide's polemical *AIDS Hysteria*, 2nd ed. (Dallas: Monument Press, 1988) provides a discussion of several imported and domestic AIDS conspiracy theories. Les Wright's "Gay Genocide as Literary Trope," in *AIDS: The Literary Response*, ed. Emmanuel S. Nelson (New York: Twayne Publishers, 1992), 50–68 offers a detailed analysis of the conspiracy notion in several novels about AIDS.

45. *Reports*, 68–74; "100,000 and Counting," *Outweek*, August 14, 1989, 38–39; *Reports*, 199.

46. *Reports*, 314, 317, 319.

47. Thorne, 27.

48. Scott Tucker, *Fighting Words*, 47–48.

49. In particular, Kramer cites Primo Levi's *Survival in Auschwitz*, trans. Stuart Woolf (New York: Summit, 1985), originally, *If This Is a Man*) and *The Drowned and the Saved*, trans. Raymond Rosenthal (New York: Summit, 1988); Hannah Arendt's *Eichmann in Jerusalem: A Report on the Banality of Evil*, rev. ed. (New York: Penguin, 1978) and Ron H. Feldman, ed. *The Jew as Pariah: Jewish Identity Politics in the Modern Age* (New York: Grove, 1978); John Boswell's *Christianity, Social Tolerance, and Homosexuality*; Ernest Becker's *Escape from Evil* (New York: Free Press, 1975); and Zygmunt Bauman's *Modernity and the Holocaust* (Cambridge, England: Polity Press, 1989).

50. *Reports*, 229; 263; 265; 287.

51. "A 'Manhattan Project' for AIDS" first appeared on the op-ed page of the *New York Times* on July 16, 1990 (*Reports*, 356–60) and "Name an AIDS High Command" on the same pages on November 15, 1992 (*Reports*, 391–97).

52. *Reports*, 384; 331; 369; 448–49.

53. Thorne, 29.

54. Ian Young, *The Stonewall Experiment: A Gay Psychohistory* (London: Cassell, 1995); Douglas Sadownick, *Sex Between Men: An Intimate History of the Sex Lives of Gay Men Postwar to Present* (San Francisco: HarperSanFrancisco, 1996).

55. Joel Shatzky, "AIDS Enters the American Theater: *As Is* and *The Normal Heart*," Nelson 131–39; Clive Barnes, "Plague, Play and Tract," review of Larry Kramer's *The Normal Heart*, *New York Post*, May 4, 1985, *New York Theatre Critics' Reviews*. New York: Critics' Theatre Reviews, 1985; D. S. Lawson, "Rage and Remembrance: The AIDS Plays," Nelson 140–154; James Miller, "Dante on Fire Island," 265–305; Michael Feingold, "Introduction," in *The Way We Live Now: American Plays and the AIDS Crisis*, ed. M. Elizabeth Osborn (New York: Theatre Communications Group, 1990), xvi, and "Messiah Complexities" review of Larry Kramer's *The Destiny of Me*, *Village Voice*, October 27, 1992, 109.

56. Clive Barnes " 'Destiny" Finds Hope in Despair," review of Larry Kramer's *The Destiny of Me*, *New York Post*, October 21, 1992; and John Simon, review of Larry Kramer's *The Destiny of Me*, *New York*, November 2, 1992, both in *New York Theatre Critics' Reviews* (New York: Critics' Theatre Reviews, 1992).

57. Philip M. Kayal, *Bearing Witness: Gay Men's Health Crisis and the Politics of AIDS* (Boulder, CO: Westview Press, 1993), 214, 215.

58. Lee Edelman, "The Plague of Discourse: Politics, Literary Theory, and 'AIDS,' " 79–92, 86, 89; and "The Mirror and the Tank: 'AIDS,' Subjectivity, and the Rhetoric of Activism," in *Homographesis: Essays in Gay Literary and Cultural Theory* (New York: Routledge, 1994), 107. As Nicholas de Jongh notes in his *Not in Front of the Audience* (New York: Routledge, 1992) about *The Normal Heart*, "The sensibilities of the great gay may be tempered by their homosexuality, but it is implausible to argue that these artists share an identity. It is no more than a conjuring trick to imagine that gay culture sweeps into existence through the naming of great homosexuals in history, when the homosexuals whom he names have a necessarily different sense of their identity, and may not even have a homosexual identity in the sense we understand it" (185).

59. John D'Emilio, "A Meaning for All Those Words: Sex Politics, History and Larry Kramer," in *We Must Love One Another or Die: The Life and Legacies of Larry Kramer*, ed. Lawrence D. Mass (New York: St. Martin's Press, 1997), 73–85.

60. David Bergman, "Larry Kramer and the Rhetoric of AIDS," in *Gaiety Transfigured: Gay Self-Representation in American Literature* (Madison, WI: University of Wisconsin Press, 1991), 122–38; Bergman alluded to Kramer's self-description as a "message queen" in a speech given in 1987 at a GMHC-sponsored forum: "I only know that at this stage of my own life, with death so palpable and continuously close, I only have time, with whatever professional authority my years of living and experience have given me, to be— a message queen. . . . I just wish that those who do call themselves artists, or those who traffic in art . . . would call themselves artists less and become message queens more" (*Reports*, 146, 147).

61. *Reports*, "We Killed Vito" 369–73; Bercovitch, *American Jeremiad*, 190.

62. Bergman, 128.

63. Richard Hofstadter, "The Paranoid Style in American Politics," in *The Fear of Conspiracy: Images of Un-American Subversion from the Revolution to the Present*, ed. David Brion Davis (Ithaca, NY: Cornell University Press, 1971), 2–9; rep. from Richard Hofstadter, *The Paranoid Style in American Politics* (New York: Alfred A. Knopf, 1964, 1965).

64. Bercovitch, 180, 181.

65. Bergman 136; Bercovitch 190–91.

NOTES TO CHAPTER FOUR

1. Charles Ortleb, "The West Street Massacre," *New York Native*, December 5–18, 1980, 4–7.

2. *AIDS and Its Metaphors* (New York: Farrar, Straus, Giroux, 1988), 94.

3. Ernest Tuveson, *Redeemer Nation: The Idea of America's Millennial Role* (Chicago: University of Chicago Press, 1968), 199. In "Sin versus Science: Venereal Disease

in Twentieth-Century Baltimore," historian Elizabeth Fee notes that an innovative "sex hygiene" curriculum for high school students during World War II employed military metaphors in discussing sex (137). Daniel M. Fox in "AIDS and American Health Polity: The History and Prospects of a Crisis of Authority" discusses President Nixon's "declaration" of a "war on cancer" in 1970 (320). In "AIDS, Gender, and Biomedical Discourse," Paula A. Treichler records Donna J. Haraway's observation in "The Biological Enterprise" that immunologists have shifted from metaphors of World War II tactical combat to postwar/ Cold War metaphors of communication and information tactics (249, n55). All three articles are found in Fee and Fox (eds.) *AIDS: The Burdens of History* (Berkeley: University of California Press, 1988). See also Ruth Bloch's *Visionary Republic: Millennial Themes in American Thought, 1756–1800* (Cambridge: Cambridge University Press, 1985) for an illuminating study of early American and Colonial apocalypticism and millennialism.

4. "The *Poz* 50." *Poz.* Aug./Sept. 1996: 62–74; John Lauritsen, *The AIDS War: Propaganda, Profiteering, and Genocide from the Medical-Industrial Complex* (New York: Asklepios, 1993), 9; Andrew Holleran, *Ground Zero* (New York: Plume, 1988), 17.

5. Scott Tucker, *Fighting Words: An Open Letter to Queers and Radicals* (London: Cassell, 1995), 7.

6. *AIDS and Its Metaphors* (New York: Farrar, Straus, Giroux, 1988), 5.

7. *Illness as Metaphor* (New York: Vintage, 1977, 1978); *AIDS and Its Metaphors*, 94.

8. Brian Patton, "Cell Wars: Military Metaphors and the Crisis of Authority in the AIDS Epidemic," in *Fluid Exchanges: Artists and Critics in the AIDS Crisis*, ed. James Miller (Toronto: University of Toronto Press, 1992), 272–86; Daniel Fox, "AIDS and the American Health Polity: The History and Prospects of a Crisis of Authority," 316–43; Sarah Schulman, "Women Need Not Apply: Institutional Discrimination in AIDS Drug Trials," in *My American History: Lesbian and Gay Life during the Reagan/Bush Years*, foreword by Urvashi Vaid (New York: Routledge, 1994), 176–79; originally published in the *Village Voice*, February 1988.

9. "The Language of War in AIDS Discourse," in *Writing AIDS: Gay Literature, Language, and Analysis*, ed. Timothy F. Murphy and Suzanne Poirer (New York: Columbia University Press, 1993), 39–53.

10. Other critical sources are worth mentioning: Simon Watney articulates two basic forms of AIDS education internationally: the Terrorist Model and the Missionary Model. In the Terrorist Model, HIV is understood as a hidden invader who must be fended off or contained; in the Missionary Model, HIV is viewed as a savage that must be converted (or controlled). The first is the more obviously military trope, although one cannot imagine the absence of a "military force" to back up the "colonialist" efforts of the latter. See Watney's " 'The Day After Hiroshima': Reflections on official British and Swedish AIDS Education Materials and Government Policies" in his collected writings, *Practices of Freedom* (Durham: Duke University Press, 1994). In a critique of Australian AIDS education, Deborah Lupton, *Moral Threats and Dangerous Desires: AIDS in the News Media*, Social Aspects of AIDS, series ed. Peter Aggleton (London: Taylor and Francis, 1994), discusses the evocation of wartime emergency in that country's "Grim Reaper" campaign. She points out that "[s]uch rhetoric not only served to position AIDS as the

enemy, against which both the tactics of one-to-one combat and full-scale military war should be used, but also to position the government in a paternal, dominant role," while according to the same language, "the Australian public was also positioned as 'the enemy' because of its complacency, apathy and ignorance" (60). This education campaign was led by the chair of the National Advisory Committee on AIDS, a single, self-described celibate, remarkably named Ita Buttrose.

11. Schulman, *My American History,* 118. David Drake's *The Night Larry Kramer Kissed Me* (New York: Anchor Books, 1992) likewise memorializes David Summers as the first AIDS activist to be arrested. See Sarah Schulman's two accounts for the *Native,* "Committee Resolves to Close Baths: Maloney Joins Anti-Gay Sellout, Gay Activist Arrested" (114–19) and "Becoming an Angry Mob in the Best Sense: Lesbians Respond to AIDS Hysteria" (120–24) in her collected essays, *My American History.* Maxine Wolfe offered her own account of coming to AIDS activism, "AIDS and Politics: Transformation of Our Movement," in *Women, AIDS & Activism* (Boston: South End Press, 1990) 233–37, originally presented as a speech at the National Gay and Lesbian Task Force Town Meeting, October 1989 in Washington, DC.

12. Rapid AIDS Mobilization, demonstration flyer (n.d.); press release, Buddy Noro, spokesperson, June 27, 1985; Steinman Papers, National Lesbian and Gay Archives, New York City.

13. See "Gay Pride Issue" of *Lavender Hill News,* a chronology of the group's efforts in 1986 and 1987, included among the Blotcher Papers of the National Lesbian and Gay Archives in New York.

14. Matthew Daniels, "Moral Majority, Inc., and the Targeting of Gays," *New York Native,* April 20–May 3, 1981, 10+; Schulman, *My American History,* 115.

15. "A Cure for A.I.D.S." Flyer, Steinman Papers, National Lesbian and Gay Archives, New York.

16. Douglas Crimp with Adam Rolston, *AIDS Demo Graphics* (Seattle: Bay Press, 1990) 26–29.

17. See Heinz Heger's first-person account of the Nazi's treatment of homosexuals in *The Men With the Pink Triangle* (Boston: Alyson Publications, 1980).

18. Lee Edelman problematized the motto Silence = Death in his deconstructive analysis, "The Plague of Discourse: Politics, Literary Theory, and 'AIDS,' " in *Homographesis: Essays in Gay Literary and Cultural Theory* (New York: Routledge, 1994), suggesting that this figurative formula inadvertently but necessarily reinforced essentialist binary categories, and concluding that "there is no available discourse on 'AIDS' that is not itself diseased" (92).

19. Crimp with Rolston, 14–15, 30–31.

20. Douglas Crimp provided a description and analysis of this installation in "AIDS: Cultural Analysis/Cultural Activism," in his book of the same title (Cambridge, MA: MIT Press, 1987), 7–13.

21. See Crimp with Rolston. Alexandra Juhasz's *AIDS TV: Identity, Community, and Alternative Video,* videography by Catherine Saalfield (Durham, NC: Duke University

Press, 1995) offers a careful analysis of the material conditions involved in the production of some of these collective efforts.

22. Crimp with Rolston, 18.

23. Crimp with Rolston, 20.

24. The "Read My Lips" poster and a discussion of its production can be found in Crimp with Rolston, 52–58.

25. Crimp with Rolston 105.

26. Tim Miller, interview, August 10, 1995.

27. *History* 281–82.

28. Lesbian Avengers, "Dyke Manifesto," Poster/broadside, Lesbian Avengers vertical file, National Lesbian and Gay Archives, New York.

29. *Lesbian Avengers Eat Fire Too*, Video, directed by Janet Baus and Su Friedrich, (New York: N.d.). Cecilia Rodríguez Milanés informs me that *comer candela* (to eat fire) is also a traditional Cuban idiom for a fighter or tough militant.

30. *Lesbian Avengers Eat Fire Too*; Schulman *My American History*, 283–87; "Summer 1994: Thirty-five Chapters and Counting," poster, Lesbian Avengers vertical file, National Lesbian and Gay Archives, New York.

31. Many of Schulman's essays and articles are collected (some in revised form) in *My American History: Lesbian and Gay Life during the Reagan/Bush Years*, hereafter cited in text as *History*. *People in Trouble* (New York: Plume, 1990); *Empathy* (New York: Plume, 1992); *Rat Bohemia* (New York: Dutton, 1995) are hereafter cited in the text. Steven Kruger's analysis in *AIDS Narratives: Gender and Sexuality, Fiction and Science* (New York: Garland Publishing, 1996) of Schulman's *People in Trouble* offers a discussion of her activist aesthetic in the context of his larger study of AIDS narratives.

32. "Esthetics and Loss," *Artforum* (Jan. 1987): 68–71.

33. Sarah Schulman, *Stage Struck: Theater, AIDS, and the Marketing of Gay America* (Durham, NC: Duke University Press, 1998).

34. Vivian Gornick, "Outside Looking In," review. of Sarah Schulman's *Rat Bohemia*, *Women's Review of Books*, February, 1996), 9.

35. Edmund White, "A Witness to Her Time," review of *Rat Bohemia*, by Sarah Schulman, *New York Times Book Review*, January 28, 1996, 31.

36. Tucker, 40, 45–47.

37. Emily Martin's *Flexible Bodies: The Role of Immunity in American Culture from the Days of Polio to the Age of AIDS* (Boston: Beacon Press, 1994) offers both a genealogy and a prospectus on martial tropes for disease:

> There are many possible reasons why people would frequently choose a militaristic image first but, when offered the chance, could come up with many different images. The omnipresence of military imagery in the media and the authority carried by information about a scientific topic are possible relevant

factors. But the kind of society and world in which different people grow up may also be important. In our interviews, all manner of people could produce military images: young people, old people, and especially aging baby boomers, who came of age during the cold war era of the 1940s and 1950s, when imagery of the body as a fortress or a castle was most vibrant. But *all* the examples that struck me as the most elaborated, vivid departures from military imagery came from people in their late teens and early twenties, people coming of age at a time when cold war assumptions are being drastically shaken and a new sensibility about how the body relates to the world may be arising. (71)

NOTES TO CHAPTER FIVE

1. Katharine Firth discusses the Protestant fantasy of the American Indians as Lost Tribes of Israel in *The Apocalyptic Tradition in Reformation Britain, 1530–1645* (Oxford: Oxford University Press, 1979), especially 161–62, 201–3. This notion persisted even after the colonial period, as evidenced by Elias Boudinot's *A Star in the West: or, A Humble Attempt to Discover the Long Lost Ten Tribes of Israel, Preparatory to Their Return to Their Beloved City, Jerusalem* (Trenton, NJ: D. Fenton, S. Hutchinson and J. Dunham, 1816) and Charles Even's *The Lost Tribes of Israel: or, The First of the Red Men* (Philadelphia: L. Johnson, 1861).

2. Kurt Rudolph, *Gnosis: The Nature and History of Gnosticism,* trans. Robert McLachlan Wilson (San Francisco: Harper & Row, 1983) is a useful and detailed guide to gnosticisms. In an excellent article, "Uses of Gender Imagery in Ancient Gnostic Texts," in *Gender and Religion: On the Complexity of Symbols,* ed. Caroline Walker Bynum, Steven Harrell, and Paula Richman (Boston: Beacon Press, 1986), 196–225, Michael A. Williams remarks that "most Gnostic sources that have survived represent forms of Jewish or Christian gnosticism, and their uses of female imagery are indeed often in striking contrast to what is normally encountered in more 'orthodox' forms of Judaism or Christianity" (197). See also Wayne A. Meeks's "The Image of the Androgyne: Some Uses of a Symbol in Earliest Christianity," *History of Religions* 13 (1974): 183–89 and Elaine Pagels' excellent *The Gnostic Gospels* (New York: Vintage, 1979).

3. There are several useful studies of Neoplatonism. A. C. Lloyd's *The Anatomy of Neoplatonism* (Oxford: Clarendon Press, 1990) offers an overview of the subject. Another examination of the subject in the context of religious mysticism is John Peter Kennedy's *Mystical Monotheism: A Study in Ancient Platonic Theology* (Hanover, NH: University Press of New England, 1991). *Neoplatonism and Islamic Thought,* ed. Parviz Morewedge (Albany: State University of New York Press, 1992), offers some parallels to Jewish mysticism. The erudition of the late O. B. Hardison is evident in his useful summary, "Platonism and Poetry," in *The New Princeton Encyclopedia of Poetry and Poetics,* ed. Alex Preminger and T. V. F. Brogan (Princeton, NJ: Princeton University Press, 1993), 912–14, offering an overview of Neoplatonism's cultural pervasiveness. See also the tenth chapter, "Interplanetary Tours: The Platonic Space Shuttle, from Plotinus to Marsilio Ficino," in I. P. Couliano's *Out of This World: Otherworldly Journeys from Gilgamesh to Albert Einstein* (Boston: Shambhala, 1991), 188–211.

4. I borrow the description of mystery as "inexhaustible intelligibility" from Catholic theologian John S. Dunne in his *A Search for God in Time and Memory* (Notre Dame, IN: University of Notre Dame Press, 1967, 1969), 7. The classic study of Kabbalah is Gershom Scholem's *On the Kabbalah and Its Symbolism*, trans. Ralph Manheim (New York: Schocken Books, 1965, 1996). See also his *Jewish Gnosticism, Merkabah Mysticism, and Talmudic Tradition* (New York: Jewish Theological Seminary of America, 1960) and *On the Mystical Shape of the Godhead: Basic Concepts in the Kabbalah*, trans. Joachim Neugroschel, ed. Jonathan Chipman (New York: Pantheon Books, 1991). A more recent development of Kabbalah scholarship both beholden to and in critique of Scholem is Moshe Idel's *Kabbalah: New Perspectives* (New Haven: Yale University Press, 1988). Harold Bloom reads Kabbalah as a precursor of his own theory of poetic influence and intertextuality in *Kabbalah and Criticism* (New York: Seabury, 1975). See also I. P. Couliano's ninth chapter, "The Seven Palaces and the Chariot of God: Jewish Mysticism from Merkabah to Kabbalah," in *Out of This World: Otherworldly Journeys from Gilgamesh to Albert Einstein* (154–87). For a discussion of Kabbalah and English Reformation apocalypticism, see Katharine Firth's *The Apocalyptic Tradition in Reformation Britain, 1530–1645*, especially 104–5 and 204–5. Two valuable studies of Kabbalah in relation to twentieth-century literary culture are R. Barbara Gitenstein's *Apocalyptic Messianism and Contemporary Jewish-American Poetry* (Albany, NY: State University of New York Press, 1986) and Robert Alter's *Necessary Angels: Tradition and Modernity in Kafka, Benjamin, and Scholem* (Cambridge, MA: Harvard University Press, 1991).

5. Brooke (Cambridge: Cambridge University Press, 1994), 7–8

6. Harold Bloom, *The American Religion: The Emergence of the Post-Christian Nation* (New York: Simon and Schuster, 1992), 31. John L. Brooke cites his debt to R. Laurence Moore's "The Occult Connection? Mormonism, Christian Science, and Spiritualism," in *The Occult in America: New Historical Perspectives*, ed. Howard Kerr and Charles L. Crow (Urbana, IL: University of Illinois Press, 1983), 137–43). For a study of English Reformation radicalism, see Christopher Hill's *The World Turned Upside Down: Radical Ideas During the English Revolution* (New York: Viking, 1972). Despite Bloom's reservations, a classic study of the Church of Jesus Christ of Latter-Day Saints is Klaus J. Hansen's *Mormonism and the American Experience* (Chicago: University of Chicago Press, 1981). An interesting companion to Brooke's study is Erich Robert Paul's *Science, Religion, and Mormon Cosmology* (Urbana, IL: University of Illinois Press, 1992). A recent study of Mormonism's assimilation into the dominant Protestant culture of the United States, an issue of concern among some gay and lesbian activists, can be found in Armand L. Mauss' *The Angel and the Beehive: The Mormon Struggle with Assimilation* (Urbana, IL: University of Illinois Press, 1994). See also Arthur Versluis, *The Esoteric Origins of the American Renaissance* (Oxford: Oxford University Press, 2001) for a discussion of the relationship between American romanticism and hermeticism.

7. *Angels in America, Part One: Millennium Approaches* (New York: Theatre Communications Group, 1992, 1993); *Angels in America, Part Two: Perestroika* (New York: Theatre Communications Group, 1992, 1994); hereafter cited in the text. The term "fabulous realism" is Sarah Schulman's in her novel *Rat Bohemia* (New York: Dutton, 1995) where the character David remarks: "No one can deny that, after all, there is something about desire that makes men treat each other like meat and love it. Goodness

and badness have nothing to do with it. Desire can't be decided. But there is also that strange combination of camaraderie in nelly machismo. It is what the literary critics would call *fabulous realism* if they weren't too stupid to notice" (58). Kushner has noted "[t]he fact that George [C. Wolfe, the plays' New York director] is gay is a plus for me. He brings a certain fabulousness to his work" (quoted in Don Shewey "Tony Kushner's Sexy Ethics: The Epic 'Angels in America' Dares to Ask the Big Question: What Does AIDS Tell Us about the Human Soul?" *Village Voice*, April 20, 1993, 29+; quote from 32) as well as characterizing David Greenspan's work and his own as "Theater of the Fabulous" (Shewey, 31). See also David Savran, "The Theatre of the Fabulous: An Interview with Tony Kushner," in *Essays on Kushner's Angels*, ed. Per Brask (Winnipeg, Manitoba: Blizzard Publishing, 1995), 129–54; Brask collects essays with an international perspective, documenting the plays' effects in Europe and Australia. Another collection of academic essays is Deborah R. Geis and Steven F. Kruger, eds., *Approaching the Millennium: Essays on* Angels in America (Ann Arbor: University Michigan Press, 1997); see also the collection of interviews, *Tony Kushner in Conversation*, ed. Robert Vorlicky (Ann Arbor: University Michigan Press, 1998).

8. Bruce Weber reports on the fierce rivalries among New York producers in their competition to have *Millennium Approaches* produced at their theaters ("A Theater Is Selected for 'Angels,'" *New York Times*, December 11, 1992, C3). An off-Broadway opening at the Joseph Papp Public Theatre was bypassed, causing further hard feelings. In signing an agreement with producers, Kushner ensured that following the Tony Awards, 800 seats each week would be available at $19.50 and $30 in addition to the standard $60, as well as the condition that a dollar from every ticket would be donated to Broadway Cares/Equity Fights AIDS (Shewey, 32).

9. Quoted in Shewey, 30.

10. John Lahr, "Early Angels," *New Yorker*, December 13, 1993, 129–33; quote from 131. Kushner quoted in Shewey, 31.

11. Brooke, 8. Jung's classic text employing alchemical tropes is *Mysterium Coniunctionis: An Inquiry into the Separation and Synthesis of Psychic Opposites in Alchemy*, 2nd ed. trans. R. F. C. Hull. Bollingen Series XX (Princeton: Princeton University Press, 1963, 1970). For discussions of Jung's appropriation of alchemical symbols, see Northrop Frye's "The Archetypes of Literature: 'Forming Fours,' 'Expanding Eyes," *Jungian Literary Criticism*, ed. Richard P. Sugg (Evanston, IL: Northwestern University Press, 1992), 21–37; Richard E. Messer's "Alchemy and Individuation in *The Magus*," Sugg, 343–51; and Gilles Quispel's "Gnosis and Culture," *C. B. Jung and the Humanities: Toward a Hermeneutics of Culture*, ed. Karin Barnaby and Pellegrino D'Acierno (Princeton, NJ: Princeton University Press, 1990), 24–35.

12. Benjamin "Theses on the Philosophy of History," in *Critical Theory Since 1965*, ed. Hazard Adams and Leroy Searle (Tallahassee, FL: University Press of Florida, 1986), 680–85; quote from 681.

13. Benjamin, 682.

14. Alter, 116.

15. I am using Robert Hodge and Gunther Kress' terminology to distinguish discourse's representational strategies (the mimetic plane) from its message strategies (the

semiosic plane). See *Social Semiotics* (Ithaca, NY: Cornell University Press, 1988), 5. Also see Rob Baker's chapter 20, "Alchemy & *Angels in America*," in *The Art of AIDS* (New York: Continuum, 1994) for a discussion of the structural homology between the two parts of the play and the alchemical process.

16. See Emile Benveniste's "The Semiology of Language," *Semiotics: An Introductory Anthology*, ed. Robert E. Innis (Bloomington, IN: Indiana University Press, 1985), 226–46 and Thomas A. Sebeok's *The Sign and Its Masters* (Austin: University Texas Press, 1979). Winfried Nöth's discussion of language codes can be found in *Handbook of Semiotics* (Bloomington, IN: Indiana University Press, 1990), 237–39. Keir Elam summarizes the position of the Prague structuralists in *The Semiotics of Theatre and Drama* (London: Methuen, 1980), 3–19. See Susanne K. Langer's discussion of ritual as symbolic transformation in *Philosophy in a New Key* (New York: Mentor, 1951). For discussions of a social semiotic theory of transformations, see Robert Hodge's Chapter 5, "Transformations," in *Literature as Discourse: Textual Strategies in English and History* (Johns Hopkins University Press, 1990), and Hodge and Gunther Kress' chapter 6, "Transformation and Time," in *Social Semiotics*, 162–203.

17. See John B. Thompson's, "Introduction," in *Language and Symbolic Power* by Pierre Bourdieu, trans. Gino Raymond and Matthew Adamson (Cambridge, MA: Harvard University Press, 1991), 1–31.

18. *American Religion*, 17.

19. Arthur Lubow, "Tony Kushner's Paradise Lost," *New Yorker*, November 30, 1992, 59–64; quote from 60.

20. Don Shewey, "Tony Kushner's Sexy Ethics," 31.

21. *Thinking*, 32.

22. *Thinking*, 223, 224.

23. *Thinking*, 16.

24. Greeley, *The Religious Imagination* (New York: Sadlier, 1981), 95. For a further discussion of sacred eros in Kabbalah mysticism, see Gershom Scholem's chapter 3, "Kabbalah and Myth" (87–117), and chapter 4, "Tradition and New Creation in the Ritual of the Kabbalists" (118–57), in *On the Kabbalah and Its Symbolism*. As Scholem's account points out, the intensity of Kabbalah mysticism could veer off into two polar directions: on the one hand, a purity cult believing that male seed discharged during nocturnal emission or masturbation created demons, and on the other the erotic antinomianism of Sabbateanism and Frankism. Moshe Idel points out a Talmudic tradition concerning the cherubim in I Kings, who are portrayed as "catalyzer[s] of human intercourse" (130). See also R. Barbara Gitenstein's discussion of sexuality and cosmic union in *Apocalyptic Messianism and Contemporary Jewish-American Poetry*, especially 63–69 and 102–3. Andrew Greeley's article "Religion and Attitudes toward AIDS Policy," *AIDS, Ethics & Religion: Embracing a World of Suffering*, ed. Kenneth R. Overbaugh, S.J. (Maryknoll, NY: Orbis Books, 1994), 223–30 correlates people's images of God with their attitudes about people with AIDS.

25. Robert Chesley, *Jerker, or The Helping Hand, Out Front: Contemporary Gay and Lesbian Plays*, ed. Don Shewey (New York: Grove, 1988) 449–91; quote from 475. *Longtime Companion*, film written by Craig Lucas, directed by Norman René (American Playhouse, 1990).

26. "Friends at Evening," *Men on Men*, ed. George Stambolian (New York: Plume, 1986), 88–113; quote from 101. Dreuilhe, *Mortal Embrace: Living with AIDS*, trans. Linda Coverdale (New York: Hill and Wang, 1988), 126.

27. An extensive queer spiritual literature has accrued since Stonewall, including: John J. McNeill, *The Church and the Homosexual*, 4th ed (Boston: Beacon Press, 1976, 1985, 1988, 1993); Letha Dawson and Virginia Ramey Mollenkott, *Is the Homosexual My Neighbor?: A Positive Christian Response*, rev. ed. (San Francisco: HarperSanFrancisco, 1978, 1994); Troy Perry, *The Lord Is My Shepherd and He Knows I'm Gay* (Austin, TX: Liberty Press, 1972); Lev Raphael, "To Be a Jew," *Wrestling with the Angel: Faith and Religion in the Lives of Gay Men*, ed. Brian Bouldrey (New York: Riverhead Books, 1995), 21–47; Michael Lowenthal, "Saying Kaddish for Peter," Bouldrey 259–63; and Christie Balka and Andy Rose, eds., *Twice Blessed: On Being Lesbian, Gay, and Jewish* (Boston: Beacon Press, 1989). In addition to this, there has grown an extensive literature of AIDS and spirituality. Michael Callen's interview with Rev. Steven Pieters in *Surviving AIDS* (New York: HarperCollins, 1990) is an interesting discussion of the role of spiritual healing (81–89). John Snow's *Mortal Fear: Meditations on Death and AIDS* (Cambridge: Cowley Publications, 1987) is an eloquent reflection by a pastor and professor. Peace activist and radical, Father Dan Berrigan, S.J. writes powerfully of his own encounters with people with AIDS in *Sorrow Built a Bridge: Friendship and AIDS* (Baltimore: Fortkamp Publishing, 1989). Andréa R. Vaucher includes a chapter on spirituality based on her interviews with culture workers in *Muses from Chaos and Ash: AIDS, Artists, and Art* (New York: Grove Press, 1993) 193–207. Richard L. Smith's *AIDS, Gays, and the American Catholic Church* (Cleveland, OH: Pilgrim Press, 1994) attempts to establish grounds for dialogue between gay activists and the Church and *AIDS, Ethics & Religion: Embracing a World of Suffering*, ed. Kenneth R. Overberg, SJ (Maryknoll, NY: Orbis Books, 1994), collects essays from a variety of perspectives including spirituality and health care.

28. New York: St. Martin's, 1994; hereafter cited in the text.

29. See Dawn Glanz's "The American West as Millennial Kingdom," *Apocalyptic Vision in America: Interdisciplinary Essays on Myth and Culture*, ed. Lois Parkinson Zamora (Bowling Green, OH: Bowling Green University Popular Press, 1982), 139–53. Robert V. Hine's *California's Utopian Colonies* (New York: W.W. Norton, 1966) examines several groups, secular and religious, that migrated to the West Coast between 1850 and 1950.

30. Quoted in Felice Picano "Shining Star," interview with Douglas Sadownick, *Bay Windows* (Boston), September 22, 1994), 20+.

31. Quoted in Robert Hopcke *Jung, Jungians, and Homosexuality* (Boston: Shambhala, 1989), 117.

32. *Men's Dreams, Men's Healing* (Boston: Shambhala, 1990), 125. See also Howard Teich's "Homovision: The Solar/Lunar Twin-Ego," in *Same-Sex Love and the Path to Wholeness*, ed. Robert Hopcke, Karin Lofthus Carrington, and Scott Wirth (Boston: Shambhala, 1993), 136–50 for a discussion of Mitch Walker's term "the double."

33. *Sex Between Men: An Intimate History of the Sex Lives of Gay Men Postwar to Present* (San Francisco: HarperSanFrancisco, 1996), 240; hereafter cited in the text.

34. *Dark Eros: The Imagination of Sadism*, 2nd ed. (Woodstock, CT: Spring Publications, 1990, 1994), 193.

35. See Odets' *In the Shadow of the Epidemic: Being HIV-Negative in the Age of AIDS* (Durham,NC: Duke University Press, 1995). Eric Rofes took up Odets' concerns in *Reviving the Tribe: Regenerating Gay Men's Sexuality and Culture in the Ongoing Epidemic* (New York: Harrington Park Press, 1996), but Gabriel Rotello is critical of both in his *Sexual Ecology: AIDS and the Destiny of Gay Men* (New York: Dutton, 1997).

36. Sadownick was responding to a passage from Judith Butler's *Bodies that Matter: On the Discursive Limits of Sex*: "To claim that discourse is formative is not to claim that it originates, causes, or exhaustively composes that which it concedes; rather, it is to claim that there is no reference to a pure body which is not at the same time a further formation of that body" (10). Sadownick may have been reacting obliquely to Butler's entire project, which is designed to throw into doubt the very stability of biological sex categories, thus seeming to subvert basic Jungian binarisms of *animus* and *anima*. Sadownick also has held polar views of semiotics and symbolism, collapsing the first into simple sign or code while elevating the latter to the status of mystery.

37. Beverley D. Zabriskie, "The Feminine: Pre- and Post-Jungian." Barnaby and D'Acierno, 267–78; quote from 276.

38. Carol Schreier Rupprecht, "Enlightening Shadows: Between Feminism and Archetypalism, Literature and Analysis." Barnaby and D'Acierno, 279–93; quote from 282, 287. Rupprecht bases some of her discussion on the ground breaking work of Annis V. Pratt. In "Spinning Among Fields: Jung, Frye, Lévi-Strauss, and Feminist Archetypal Theory" (Sugg, 153–66), Pratt discussed her examination of British and American women's novels from the eighteenth through the twentieth centuries tracing initiatory motifs, the rebirth quest or journey. See also Andrew Samuels' "Beyond the Feminine Principle" (Barnaby and D'Acierno 294–306), which discusses the problematics of Jung's theory of opposites and notion of contrasexuality. He is usefully prosaic by distinguishing sex and gender and by insisting that:

The notion of difference . . . can help us in the discussion about gender—not innate opposites that lead us to create an unjustified psychological division expressed in lists of antithetical qualities, each list yearning for the other so as to become whole. Not what differences between women and men there are, or have always been. (If we pursue that, we end up captured by our captivation and obsession with myth and with the eternal, the burdensome part of the legacy from Jung that I mentioned earlier.) But rather the fact, image, and social reality of difference itself—what difference is like, what the experience of difference is like. Not what a woman *is* but what being a woman is *like*. Not the archetypal structuring of woman's world but woman's personal experience in today's world. Not the meaning of a woman's life but her experience of her life. Each person remains a man or a woman, but what that means to each becomes immediate and relative, and hence capable of generational expansion and cultural challenge. All the time, the question of "masculine" and "feminine" remains in suspension—the bliss of now knowing. (300)

Samuels also interrogates the Jungian notion of heterosexuality as something innate and fundamental. Finally, he proposes that "anatomy is a metaphor for the richness and potential of the 'other'" (301), affirming the figurative character of gender.

39. Paul Kugler, "The Unconscious in a Postmodern Depth Psychology, " (Barnaby and D'Acierno, 307–18). See also the conclusion to Ricoeur's *The Symbolism of Evil*, trans. Emerson Buchanan (Boston: Beacon Press, 1967), 347–57. Kugler's use of the term "deeper" is admittedly problematic in that it imposes a vertical (and implicitly hierarchical) figure of speech onto a representation of consciousness. See also Michael Vannoy Adams' "Deconstructive Philosophy and Imaginal Psychology: Comparative Perspectives on Jacques Derrida and James Hillman" (Sugg, 231–48), which finds both Hillman's revision of Jungianism and Derrida's critique of Lévi-Strauss' structuralism remarkably similar.

40. See David Miller's comments on Jung and totalitarianism in "Jung and Postmodernism Symposium" (Barnaby and D'Acierno, 331–40; quote from 334), a conversation among Miller, Edward S. Casey, James Hillman, and Paul Kugler.

41. See "An Other Jung and An Other..." (Barnaby and D'Acierno 325–29); quote from 328. In the same article Miller confronts Jung's own divided personality. He cleverly explains the exchange of the semiotic order with the symbolic order this way:

First, Lacan fell off Freud's horse into Saussure's ditch, and signifiers took primacy over significations. Then, Kristeva fell off Lacan's horse and restressed the imaginary over the symbolic, noting that semiotic sign language emanates from instinctual drives and primary processes, whereas symbolic perspectives assimilate psyche's images to secondary process, predicative synthesis, and judgment. (328)

His reading of the semiotic/symbolic switch has direct relevance to the issue of authoritarianism, religious or otherwise:

But if a semiotician were asked today whether the fundamentalist discourse of Jerry Falwell were symbolic or semiotic, there would be no hesitation. It is symbolic: that is, it refers with semantic confidence to idolatrously believed-in contents taken literally. Today Christian literalism and Jungian fundamentalism are symbolic. They have become a knowing. But what Jung called symbolic, and recommended for the soul, is not this knowing. It is the paratactic, "gappy," unknowing that is today called semiotic. (328)

Like the ancient "knowing" or *gnosis* of gnosticism, belief in "pure" experiences (like apocalyptic visions) invites authoritarianism.

42. Miller, 329. In the "Jung and Postmodernism Symposium" Miller was able to amplify on these comments in a way that reflects on my reading of Sadownick's "impurity" resulting from his naive fiction of "purity":

None of us is going to get away from being premodern, naively realistic, instinctual, or biological. We are going to be that way from time to time. We are going to be idolatrous. We are going to be ideological. We are going to make mistakes. We are going to substantialize. We are going to place our meanings in ego. We are going to use words. It seems to me one beauties of Jung's vision is expressed in his use of the language of alchemy. One of the alchemists' dicta for their work was *solve et coagula*, dissolve and coagulate, dissolve again and coagulate again. This implies that any idea we have coagulated will ultimately dissolve, but that another idea will emerge from the dissolution. All our ideas will fail us. But that is a part of the alchemy in which all of us are participants. (336)

43. Peggy Phelan, *Unmarked: The Politics of Performance* (New York: Routledge, 1993), 178.

44. Mauss (Urbana: University of Illinois Press, 1994), 4–5.

45. Mauss, 60.

46. Rauch, "Beyond Oppression," *Beyond Queer: Challenging Gay Left Orthodoxy*, ed. Bruce Bawer (New York: Free Press, 1996), 119–27; quote from 126–27.

47. See also Jonathan Freedman, "Angels, Monsters, and Jews: Instersections of Queer and Jewish Identity in Kushner's *Angels in America*," *PMLA* 113, no. 1 (Jan. 1998): 90–102.

48. Seidman, in *Fear of a Queer Planet: Queer Politics and Social Theory*, ed. Michael Warner (Minneapolis, MN: University of Minnesota Press, 1993), 105–42; quote from 106.

49. Seidman, 137.

50. Seidman, 137.

51. See Stoddard's *For The Pleasure of His Company: An Affair of the Misty City* with an introduction by Roger Austen (San Francisco: Gay Sunshine Press, 1987), as well as Roger Austen's "Stoddard's Little Tricks in *South Sea Isles*," in *Essays on Gay Literature*, ed. Stuart Kellogg (New York: Harrington Park Press, 1985). A more complete treatment of Stoddard's life can be found in Austen's biography of the writer, *Genteel Pagan: The Double Life of Charles Warren Stoddard* (Amherst: University Massachusetts Press, 1991). For a discussion of Melville, see Robert K. Martin's *Hero, Captain, and Stranger: Male Friendship, Social Critique, and Literary Form in the Sea Novels of Herman Melville* (Chapel Hill, NC: University of North Carolina Press, 1986). Martin associates Melville's homo-utopian politics with those of Whitman, whom he discusses in *The Homosexual Tradition in American Poetry* (Austin: University Texas Press, 1979).

52. See Robert Aldrich, *The Seduction of the Mediterranean: Writing, Art, and Homosexual Fantasy* (New York: Routledge, 1993); Byrne R. S. Fone, "This Other Eden: Arcadia and the Homosexual Imagination," in *Essays on Gay Literature*, ed. Stuart Kellogg (New York: Harrington Park Press, 1985), 13–34. See also Fone's discussion of other utopian traditions in gay writing by Whitman, Bayard Taylor, and E. M. Forster in "The New Chivalry: Poetry and Pornography," a chapter in his *A Road to Stonewall:*

Male Homosexuality and Homophobia in English and American Literature (New York: Twayne, 1995).

53. Thomas E. Yingling, "Homosexuality and Utopian Discourse in American Poetry," with an introduction by Robyn Wiegman, in *Breaking Bounds: Whitman and American Cultural Studies*, ed. Betsy Erkkila and Jay Grossman (Oxford: Oxford University Press, 1996), 135–46; quote from 146; Jeffrey Weeks, "The Fabians and Utopia," *Against Nature: Essays on History, Sexuality and Identity* (London: Rivers Oram Press, 1991). Robert K. Martin discusses this source of Forster's novel in "Edward Carpenter and the Double Structure of *Maurice*," Kellogg 35–46.

54. "The Road to Utopia," ed. Bawer, 16–19.

55. *Fighting Words: An Open Letter to Queers and Radicals* (London: Cassell, 1995) 57–58.

NOTES TO AFTERWORD

1. "A Pneumonia That Strikes Gay Males" was published in the *San Francisco Chronicle* on June 6, 1981 (page 4). Journalist Randy Shilts would provide leading coverage of the epidemic's early years and would become a vocal critic of the ways that California's gay press initially failed to cover it. See Roger Streitmatter, *Unspeakable: The Rise of the Gay and Lesbian Press in America* (Boston: Faber and Faber, 1995), 243–75.

2. See Barry Brummett, *Contemporary Apocalyptic Rhetoric* (New York: Praeger, 1991) for his use of Kenneth Burke's term to describe the way that "people turn to writing and speaking to help them formulate symbolic structures through which they confront their everyday, lived problems and possibilities" (10).

3. Lee Quinby, *Anti-Apocalypse: Exercises in Genealogical Criticism* (Minneapolis, MN: University of Minnesota Press, 1994), 162; William Haver, *The Body of This Death: Historicity and Sociality in the Time of AIDS* (Stanford: Stanford University Press, 1996), 52.

4. Francis Fukuyama, *The End of History and the Last Man* (New York: Free Press, 1992). See also Richard G. Mitchell, Jr., *Dancing at Armageddon: Survivalism and Chaos in Modern Times* (Chicago: Chicago University Press, 2001) for a discussion of right-wing apocalypticism. Ron Powers, "The Apocalypse of Adolescence," *Atlantic Monthly*, March 2002, 58–74, employs the trope by equating nihilism with an apocalyptic mentality in his exploration of adolescent violence.

5. Robert Jay Lifton, "Giving Meaning to Survival," *Chronicle of Higher Education*, September 28, 2001, B8–B9; Michael Hardt and Antonio Negri, *Empire* (Cambridge, MA: Harvard University Press, 2000); Benjamin Barber, *Jihad vs. McWorld: How Globalism and Tribalism Are Reshaping the World* (New York: Ballantine, 1996); Valerie Strauss and Emily Wax, "Where Two Worlds Collide: Muslim Schools Face Tension of Islamic, U.S. Views," *Washington Post*, February 25, 2002, A1+.

6. Laurie Garrett, *Betrayal of Trust: The Collapse of Global Public Health* (New York: Hyperion, 2001); and *The Coming Plague: Newly Emerging Diseases in a World Out of Balance* (New York: Penguin, 1995).

7. See Mirko D. Grmek, *History of AIDS: Emergence of a Modern Pandemic*, trans. Russell C. Maulitz and Jacalyn Duffin (Princton, NJ: Princeton University Press, 1990); *Outbreak*, dir. Wolfgang Petersen (Warner Brothers, 1995); Barton Gellman, "The Belated Global Response to AIDS in Africa," *Washington Post*, July 5, 2000, A1+, and Jon Jeter, "South Africa's Advances Jeopardized by AIDS," *Washington Post*, July 6, 2000, A1+; "Mugabe and the church continue attack on gays and lesbians," *International Gay and Lesbian Human Rights Commission Home Page*, March 1996, http://www.iglhrc.org/world/africa/Zimbabwe1996Mar.html (accessed March 1, 2002).

8. Robin Gorna, *Vamps, Virgins and Victims: How Can Women Fight AIDS?* (New York: Cassell, 1996), 348. On AIDS pharmaceutical marketing, see Jayson Blair, "Healthy Skepticism and the Marketing of AIDS," *New York Times*, August 5, 2001. Andrew Sullivan, "When Plagues End: Notes on the Twilight of an Epidemic," *Independent on Sunday*, February 16, 1997: 7–11, quotation from 11; David Román, "Understanding HIV Negatives and the Problem of Seroconversion," *Wilde*, Aug./Sept. 1995: 53–56; Walt Odets, *In the Shadow of the Epidemic: Being HIV-Negative in the Age of AIDS* (Durham, NC: Duke University Press, 1995), 100; Eric Rofes, *Reviving the Tribe: Regenerating Gay Men's Sexuality and Culture in the Ongoing Epidemic* (New York: Harrington Park Press, 1996). Alex P. Kellogg, " 'Safe Sex Fatigue' Grows among Gay Students," *Chronicle of Higher Education*, January 18, 2002 documents the extent of this change; the title also suggests that it is "crisis fatigue" that partly underlies the erosion in adherence to safer sex practices, perhaps related to the exhaustion of apocalyptic urgency.

9. Buchanan is nothing if not persistent in preaching this jeremiad. See his *The Death of the West: How Dying Populations and Immigrant Invasions Imperil Our Country and Civilization* (New York: Thomas Dunne Books, 2001) in which he cites declining birth rates among Euro-Americans, the growth of immigration into the United States, an anti-Western multiculturalism promoted by the intelligentsia, and the defection of ruling elites to the idea of global government as causes for our decline.

10. Richard L. Smith's *AIDS, Gays, and the American Catholic Church* (Cleveland, OH: Pilgrim Press, 1994), offers a nuanced discussion of Catholic attitudes on sexuality and homosexuality; see also Andrew Greeley, *Religion as Poetry* (New Brunswick, NJ: Transaction Publishers, 1995). Chris Bull and John Gallagher, *Perfect Enemies: The Religious Right, the Gay Movement, and the Politics of the 1990s* (New York: Crown, 1996) analyze the way that religious conservatives have used queers to make political hay. Fred Phelps documents his own venom on his Web site: *The Westboro Baptist Church Home Page*, http://www.godhatesfags.com. For the Southern Poverty Law Center's report on hate broadcasting, see James Latham, "From America, with Hate," *Intelligence Report*, Fall 2001: 56–58.

11. Daniel Harris, *The Rise and Fall of Gay Culture* (New York: Hyperion, 1997).

12. Bloom's discussions can be found in his 1992 *The American Religion: The Emergence of the Post-Christian Nation* (New York: Simon & Schuster, 1992), and more recently in *Omens of Millennium: The Gnosis of Angels, Dreams, and Resurrection* (New York: Riverhead Books, 1996).

13. "Mitch Walker: Visionary Love, The Magickal Gay Spirit-Power," in *Gay Soul: Finding the Heart of Gay Spirit and Nature with Sixteen Writers, Healers, Teachers, and*

Visionaries, ed. Mark Thompson (San Francisco: HarperSanFrancisco, 1994), 210–36; Judy Grahn, *Another Mother Tongue: Gay Words, Gay Worlds*, rev. ed. (Boston: Beacon Press, 1984, 1990), 4–5. See Hay's "A Separate People Whose Time Has Come," ed. Thompson, 279–91. Hay's early theorizing about homosexual people figures in Sadownick's *Sex Between Men: An Intimate History of the Sex Lives of Gay Men Postwar to Present* (San Francisco: Harper, 1996), 58–60; and in Young's *The Stonewall Experiment: A Gay Psychohistory* (London: Cassell, 1995), 48–49.

14. Theologian David Tracy describes limit-situations as referring to "two basic kinds of existential situation: either those 'boundary' situations of guilt, anxiety, sickness and the recognition of death as one's own destiny, or those situations called 'ecstatic experiences'—intense joy, love, reassurance, creation. All genuine limit-situations refer to those experiences, both positive and negative, wherein we both experience our own human limits (limit-to) as our own as well as recognize, however haltingly, some disclosure of a limit-of our experience" (*Blessed Rage for Order: The New Pluralism in Theology* [New York, Seabury, 1975], 105). Among the negative experiences that Tracy has in mind are those that make us aware of our "finitude, contingency, mortality, alienation or oppression" (*The Analogical Imagination: Christian Theology and the Culture of Pluralism* [New York, Crossroad, 1981], 60). Langdon Gilkey urges that "the phenomenological character of these experiences has a qualitatively different tone from our experience of the system of finite things we investigate and call the natural world or the universe. Inevitably, there appears in this dimension a quality of the unconditioned, of the infinite, of transcendence, of the ultimate, even of what we are calling the 'holy' or the 'sacred,' a quality which does not derive from natural, finite things taken either separately or in systematic interrelations, and which in turn manifests itself as the basis or foundation of the being and the value of those things" (*Naming the Whirlwind: The Renewal of God-Language* [New York: Bobbs-Merrill, 1969], 312), in a phrase, a dimension of ultimacy.

15. Reza Abdo, quoted in Andréa R. Vaucher, *Muses from Chaos and Ash: AIDS, Artists, and Art* (New York: Grove Press, 1993), 198–99; Mark Matousek, "Savage Grace," in *In the Company of My Solitude: American Writing from the AIDS Pandemic*, ed. Marie Howe and Michael Klein (New York: Persea, 1995), 62–81.

16. Pages 21–35.

17. The most substantial of these is the last, theologian Mary E. Hunt's article on Queer Theology (59–60).

18. See the editor's comments on page 4. Many of both the feature articles and the reviews touch on topics related to religion or spirituality, Western, Eastern, and indigenous American.

19. See Rosenau (Princeton, NJ: Princeton University Press, 1992), 6, 148–52.

20. Andrew Wernick, "Post-Marx: Theological Themes in Baudrillard's *America*," *Shadow of Spirit: Postmodernism and Religion*, ed. Philippa Berry and Andrew Wernick (New York: Routledge, 1992), 57–71.

21. Jean Baudrillard, *The Illusion of the End*, trans. Chris Turner (Stanford: Stanford University Press, 1994), 22, 51, 117.

22. In *A Search for God in Time and Memory* (Notre Dame, IN: University of Notre Dame Press, 1967, 1969), Dunne further asserted that each person is "inexhaustible, incapable of being reduced to a single standpoint or to any sum of standpoints" (7). In his earlier *The City of the Gods: A Study in Myth and Mortality* (Notre Dame, IN: University of Notre Dame Press, 1965) Dunne had distinguished "mystery" as not being unsolved problems (the positivist inclination) but as an "inexhaustible source of soluble problems" (4).

23. Carl Raschke, "Fire and Roses, or the Problem of Postmodern Religious Thinking," ed. Berry and Wernick, 93–108.

24. Audre Lorde, "Uses of the Erotic: The Erotic as Power," *Sexuality and the Sacred: Sources for Theological Reflection*, ed. James B. Nelson and Sandra P. Longfellow (Louisville, KY: Wesminster/John Knox Press, 1994), 75–79.

25. Harrison and Heyward, "Pain and Pleasure: Avoiding the Confusions of Christian Tradition in Feminist Theory," ed. Nelson and Longfellow, 131–48. See also Carter Heyward's *Touching Our Strength: The Erotic as Power and the Love of God* (San Francisco: HarperSanFrancisco, 1989), in which she urges that "such sexual expression generates more energy (rather than less, apologies to Freud) for passionate involvement in the movements for justice in the world. Lovemaking turns us simultaneously *into* ourselves and *beyond* ourselves" (4).

26. See Carrington's "Women Loving Women: Speaking the Truth in Love," in *Same-Sex Love and the Path to Wholeness*, ed. Robert Hopcke, Karin Loftus Carrington, and Scott Wirth (Boston: Shambhala, 1993), 88–109. Carrington also employs an alchemical trope derived from Jung: "The individuation process of a woman in love with another woman is clearly an alchemical one: they repeat the whole process of creating themselves, return to the original perfection of their true, instinctive natures, and redeem themselves and their world through reunion. The wounding of premature separation, both archetypally and personally, can then be healed" (92).

27. Calu Lester and Larry Saxxon, "AIDS in the Black Community: The Plague, the Politics, the People," in *AIDS: Principles, Practices, and Politics*, ed. Inge B. Corless and Mary Pittman-Lindeman. Reference Edition, Series in Death Education, Aging, and Health Care (New York: Hemisphere Publishing, 1989), 517–22, quotation from 518; W. C. Champion, *The Black Church and AIDS* (Glenn Heights, TX: 1991); Susan Palmer, *AIDS as an Apocalyptic Metaphor in North America* (Toronto: University of Toronto Press, 1997), 105–8; "CDC: Minorities represent more than half of new AIDS cases among gay men," *Cable News Network Home Page*, January 13, 2000, http://www.cnn.com/2000/HEALTH/AIDS/01/13/minorities.aids.02/ (accessed March 1, 2002).

28. These voices have been gathered, for example, in Brian Bouldrey's *Wrestling with the Angel: Faith and Religion in the Lives of Gay Men* (New York: Riverhead, 1995), Mark Thompson's *Gay Soul: Finding the Heart of Gay Spirit and Nature with Sixteen Writers, Healers, Teachers, and Visionaries* (San Francisco: HarperSanFrancisco, 1994), Will Roscoe's *Queer Spirits: A Gay Men's Myth Book* (Boston: Beacon Press, 1995), and perhaps the most interesting collection, because it includes a range of male sexualities, Björn Krondorfer's *Men's Bodies, Men's Gods: Male Identities in a (Post-) Christian Culture* (New York: New York University Press, 1996).

29. Raschke, 99, 105

30. Bernard McGinn, "Introduction: Apocalyptic Spirituality," *Apocalyptic Spirituality: Treatises and Letters of Lactantius, Adso of Montier-en-Der, Joachim of Fiore, the Franciscan Spirituals, Savonarola* (New York: Paulist Press, 1979) 1–16; quotations from 3, 8.

31. Doty, "Is There A Future?" ed. Howe and Klein, 3–12; quotation from 6–7; Sontag, *AIDS and Its Metaphors* (New York: Farrar, Straus, Giroux, 1988), 87, 88.

32. Matousek, *Sex, Death, and Enlightenment: A True Story* (New York: Riverhead Books, 1996), 37–39;

33. Thompson, "Andrew Harvey: Rebirth through the Wound," *Gay Soul: Finding the Heart of Gay Spirit and Nature* (San Francisco: Harper, 1994), 47–63.

34. Andrew Harvey and Mark Matousek, *Dialogues with a Modern Mystic* (New York: Quest Books, 1994) 28.

35. Quinby, xiii.

36. John Milton, *Areopagitica*.

Index